A

18th CENTURY I   ᴄᴛᴏʀ.

William Perfect of West Malling

Shirley Burgoyne Black

Darenth Valley Publications

1995

Published in 1995 by
Darenth Valley Publications
33 Tudor Drive
Otford
Sevenoaks
Kent
TN14 5QP

A catalogue record for this book is available from the
British Library

ISBN 0 9507334 7 4

Typeset by Friary Music Services
142 Friary Road
London
SE15 5UW

Contents

Acknowledgments

I am grateful to the Centre for Kentish Studies for permission to reproduce Almeria's name scratched on glass and the signature of William Perfect. The portrait of William Perfect as a young man is based on a print in the Royal College of Physicians. The portrait of William Perfect as an older man was photographed in the Masonic Museum and Library at Canterbury, where I received a kind welcome and much friendly encouragement in this project.

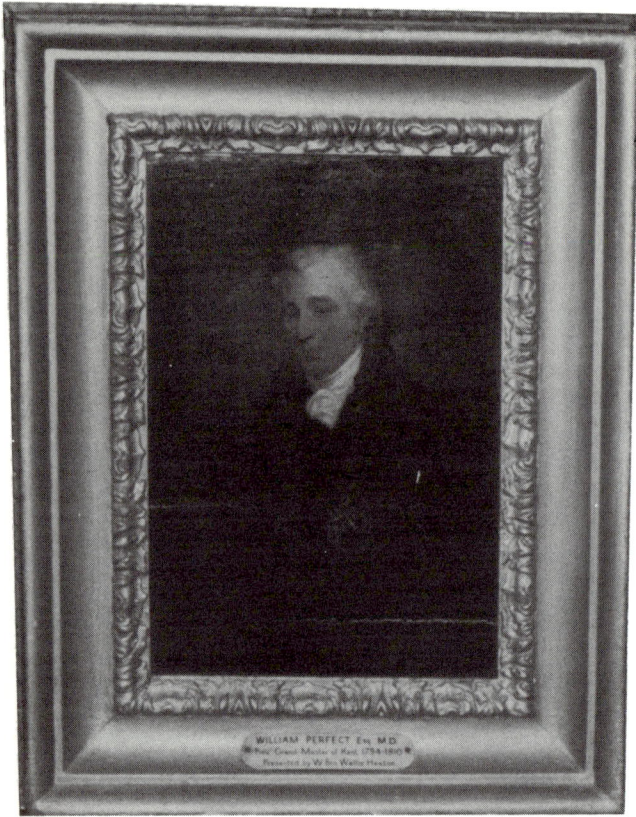

Portrait of William Perfect in the Masonic Museum, Canterbury.

Foreword

Dr William Perfect of West Malling is not unknown to historiography. As someone who, in his day, was a relatively well known 'mad-doctor', he now receives mentions in histories of insanity, and he is also encountered in the history of midwifery, an area in which he became something of a specialist before turning to insanity. Dr Perfect is also found, later in his life, in the records of freemasonry, where he can be said to have attained his highest social distinction. The present work, an attempt at a fuller biography of this eighteenth century figure than has yet appeared, developed out of a paper given at a Kent History Seminar in Otford on 17 September 1994.

It was as a practising doctor with special interests that William Perfect himself wrote, in his middle years, on both midwifery and insanity, and it is these works which are not infrequently referred to, in histories of these fields. Hunter and Macalpine's *Three Hundred Years of Psychiatry* (1963) contains a brief introduction to Perfect and his two main works, and quotes, in part, four of the cases encountered by Perfect. Herbert R. Spencer's *History of British Midwifery from 1650 to 1800* (1927) describes him as 'a highly esteemed surgeon of West Malling'.

Fairly early on in his life Perfect became a freemason, and in 1795 was elected Provincial Grand Master of the Provincial Grand Lodge of Kent. A brother freemason, Sydney Pope, made him in part the subject of an article which appeared in *Ars Quatuor Coronatorum: Transactions of Quatuor Coronati Lodge*, London, in 1939, and more recently another freemason, Roland A. Spiller, has also written on Perfect, under the title, 'William Perfect MD of West Malling, Kent, 1737-1809: Provincial Grand Master of Kent 1795-1809'. Both these articles make use of nine volumes of MSS left by William Perfect, covering the years 1754 to 1773, and now in the Masonic Museum and Library at Canterbury. I am extremely grateful to Roland Spiller for drawing my attention to this masonic material.

More unexpectedly, an Australian poet, A. W. Gaudron, in a slim volume of 1993, *Concision and Precision*, containing both poetry and prose, devotes nearly 30 pages to casting doubt on whether all the cases of insanity described by Perfect were actually his, or were 'concocted patients, ripped from the fictional cards of Dr Smollett':

I have estimated that, of his one hundred-odd patients listed in the *Annals*, perhaps 85% may have been real and — actually his. The rest seem to be very clever concoctions of literary mishmash, produced in the artificial and stinted mode of 'scholarship' which can be found in an abundant number of 18th century authors.

The figure of 85% is surely something of a give-away here. If Perfect was able to write about such a high proportion of 'real' patients, why should he have risked his reputation for a mere 15% of 'concoctions'? If some of his cases resemble those found in Smollett, one can conclude, without surprise, that two doctors, living and working around the same time, encountered similar cases. As for an 'artificial and stinted mode of "scholarship" : such a phrase can only have been written in ignorance of the educated and literary person which Perfect, like Smollett himself, both doctor and writer, undoubtedly was.

Clearly, William Perfect was and is capable of arousing interest in many quarters. While not assessing him as a doctor, in which role he seems to have been firmly of his time, practising therapies such as blood-letting, purging and control of the diet, which would stabilise the body seen in terms of Galen's humours, this biography is an attempt to give as full an account as is now possible of a many-sided and much esteemed man.

Part I: THE MAN

Chapter 1

From Birth to Obituary

William Perfect may have been a man with Kentish roots, although he was not born in Kent. If we knew why his father became vicar of East Malling, in 1742, we might have the answer to the puzzle. There was a Reverend Caleb Perfect, or Parfect, in Rochester earlier in the century, credited with having laid down the regulations for the City's poorhouse. The name Perfect could be an anglicised Huguenot one, from the French 'parfait'. But it could also go back to Norman times, and be a Latinised form of the old English 'parfit'. William Perfect does not appear ever to have attempted to draw up his genealogy, and indeed, he seems to have scorned genealogical research as, frequently, no more than boasting. But he was a handsome man, with an aquiline, slightly beaked nose, and one could, perhaps, see French ancestry in that.

His immediate family seems to have originated in what could be described as middle England. In some lines he wrote in one of his MS books he claimed Oxford as his native town, in a fairly general way, but in another verse, written as a rebus, he spells out Bicester as the place where he was born:

> What we frequently do when our money we spend, (buy)
> And when to the poor our assistance we lend, (cess — the poor rate)
> Which, joined with the half of a word for the earth, (ter-ra)
> At once will discover the place of my birth. (Bi-ces-ter)

One has to presume, of course, that he was there writing about himself, and that this was not penned for someone else. Perfect was an easy versifier, and was always happy to provide a friend with a set of verses. Bicester, rather than Oxford, seems to be confirmed as the place where his early years were spent, by some lines in his poem 'September'. As the autumn comes on, says Perfect,

> To B — 's shades resorts my youthful muse...
> To B — 's shades, where first my muse began

To wake the poet, and inform the man.

Otherwise, we know little about his youth. In 1745 the *Gentleman's Magazine* announced the appointment of his father, the Revd William Perfect, to the curacy of East Malling, although when he died, in the summer of 1757, he was to be described as its vicar. The Revd William Perfect was apparently buried in the church itself, as had been his own father, also called William, on his death two years earlier. The memorial inscription over the Perfect vault in the churchyard, however, erected some years later by William Perfect of West Malling, describes the grandfather as 'late of the city of Worcester'.

The vicar's widow, William's mother, Mrs Sarah Perfect, outlived her husband by some years. On 9 June 1759, two years after his death, she was admitted into Bromley College, which appears to have been the oldest foundation for clergymen's widows in England, founded in 1666 by John Warner, the then Bishop of Rochester. Although its inmates seem to have come from many parts of England, the widows of Kentish clerics were perhaps given a preference in what was clearly quite a prestigious establishment: 1759 saw the admission also of Mrs Ann Oare, the widow of the rector of Ditton and Allington, and of Mrs Elizabeth Soan, widow of the vicar of the Isle of Grain and of Hartlip, while in 1760 Dame Mary Burdett, whose husband, Sir Hugh Burdett, Bt, had been vicar of Newington, came to reside there. William Perfect, in his MSS, occasionally mentions a visit to Bromley, which was probably made for the purpose of going to see his mother. Indeed, a visit in 1760 seems to have inspired the lines which he headed 'Wrote in one of the Windows of Bromley College'. The atmosphere of the College, as Perfect describes it —

> Here sacred silence lulls the soul to rest,
> And meek-eyed peace bestows her virtuous quest,
> Religion, decked in the white robes of truth

— seems to have been very much that of a convent, and one wonders if all the vicars' widows were quite as meek-eyed as Perfect describes them. His mother lived there for ten years, her burial entry, in the register of Bromley parish church, dated 26 June 1769, describing her as a 'widow of the college'.

The first date in William Perfect's life which can be established beyond doubt is that of his apprenticing, in November 1749, to William Everred, a surgeon, of London. The young Perfect was indentured for seven years, on payment of a premium of £30. This was the normal procedure for anyone wishing to become a surgeon — an ordinary practising doctor — at this time. Irvine Loudon, in his fascinating and well researched book, *Medical Care and the General Practitioner 1750-1850*, has calculated that 62% of doctors at this time came from a medical background, and that the clergy formed the next most numerous category of parents.

Loudon describes the typical surgeon, or surgeon apothecary, as a grammar school boy, who had left school at 12 or 15, with some Latin, and often a smattering of Greek, to take up an apprenticeship to a surgeon. This, says Loudon, was 'for the majority, the full extent of his general and medical education. But from mid-century an increasing number proceeded to a further period of medical instruction, which could, for example, include a year or more at a provincial hospital as a pupil of one of the surgeons, followed by a further year in London attending lectures and walking the wards of the hospitals as well as attending private courses on various medical subjects. Such instruction was apt to be haphazard. There was no official syllabus and no examination.' This, in fact, provides an excellent summary of what appears to have been the medical training of William Perfect. At the end of his apprenticeship, and when he had made his choice of where to settle, the surgeon would be licensed to practise under an Act of 1511, which provided for the bishop of the diocese to license all the surgeons (and incidentally all the midwives too) living within his see. In Kent, the licensing authority was either the Archbishop of Canterbury, or the Bishop of Rochester. William Perfect, therefore, when he finally settled at West Malling, would have been licensed by the Bishop of Rochester, obtaining a certificate signed by three other local doctors, and by the bishop or his surrogate. This would vouch for his ability as a surgeon, as well as for his being 'well affected to his Majesty King George and the present Government in Church and State' — subversion in the profession was firmly discouraged.

However, before we move on to the stage in William Perfect's career when he had completed what in effect amounted to a wholly practical training, we must pause for a moment to consider the seven years which it was intended he should spend in an apprenticeship with William Everred in London. London was a good choice because it offered, as Irvine Loudon says, the opportunity to become a pupil of a surgeon at one of the many London hospitals, or to attend one or more of the courses of lectures which they sometimes gave. There is good evidence that William Perfect availed himself of these opportunities.

We know, for example, that he attended lectures given by a London doctor who specialised in obstetrics, or midwifery, as it was called then, and from the closeness of their acquaintance can probably assume also that he accompanied him round the wards. The doctor in question was

Colin Mackenzie, a Scot, whom the reference books usually show as active
in Edinburgh. But Loudon's book happens to mention another surgeon-
apprentice, Richard Smith, of Warminster and Bristol, who, in London
in the 1760s, 'studied surgery under Joseph Else and midwifery under
Colin Mackenzie'. Dr Mackenzie was clearly a doctor who left his mark
on students: among the papers relating to Richard Smith is one noting
that Mackenzie had reproved the apprentice for going to a midwifery case
in a scarlet cloak with a sword, which was apparently fashionable attire
among medical students of the time, saying that it was 'inappropriate to
be going to bring a person into the world with a weapon intended to send
a person out of it'. Perfect must have come to know Mackenzie well, for
his book on midwifery, which went into three editions, contains numerous letters exchanged with Mackenzie, before the older doctor's death in
1775, in which they discuss some of the cases encountered by Perfect.
Irvine Loudon concludes that the talented and enthusiastic student could
find for himself a medical education which was reasonably comprehen-
sive, and that 'with this behind him he could enter practice with some
confidence and pride'. From the evidence available it seems possible to say
that William Perfect in his time was just such a student, talented and
enthusiastic, and that he, too, had confidence and pride in his abilities, a
confidence which was not misplaced.

However, although William is noted as having entered on a seven-year
apprenticeship with a London surgeon in 1749, we find him in 1754 in
Dartford, Kent. Some surgeon-apprenticeships were, in fact, for only five
years, and it is possible that William Perfect's term was reduced, particularly if he felt that his master had no more to teach him. Certainly, his
presence in Dartford seems to provide fairly conclusive evidence that his
apprenticeship had come to an end, and he may have been occupying a
temporary post there as an assistant to another surgeon, while he looked
about him for a suitable place to settle. Loudon points out that surgeons
were often the sons of surgeons, who would, in the natural course of
things, take over their father's practice. William Perfect, as the son of a
clergyman, had no such place comfortably waiting for him, although it
was probably the fact that his father held the living of East Malling which
encouraged him to look for a practice in this part of Kent.

Although it is not altogether clear why he should have come to
Dartford, where he perhaps spent two or three years, we do know that one
of the things he was doing there was writing poetry: one of the earliest in
date of the poems in his MSS is entitled, 'Wrote on a certain Bench at
Dartford'; it begins: 'To this cool shade I oft retreat', and it ends:

Regardless both of praise and blame,
Amusement all my end and game,
As here I rest unknown to fame,
Quite unconcerned when Judgment sits,
And I am damned by Dartford Wits.

This is clearly dated 25 June 1754, and it seems, from its tone, to have been written by someone, perhaps a little lonely, who has only recently come to a place, and who is prepared to cock a snook at its inhabitants.

But William Perfect was of too gregarious a nature to remain lonely for long, and he soon made friends in Dartford, particularly, one must assume, with the Williams family, since he was to keep up a lively correspondence with one member of it, Sarah Williams, for some years. Sarah, or Sally, as she was often called, was very possibly a much younger acquaintance or even a relative, educated and vivacious, an eighteenth-century girl of the type epitomised by John Wilkes' daughter, Polly. The following lines, headed 'Extempore on a young lady's ruff', were addressed to her by Perfect in July 1756:

Now Sally, now, I mean to chide
That little foolish bag of pride
That does below your chin appear,
And at your fancy wildly glare!
Such white (now my advice receive)
To hide did Nature never give.
If you would give me bliss enough,
Then straight discard the flimsy ruff!

By the time this was written the young doctor was already a married man, with one child, a daughter, Elizabeth, and another shortly to follow. It seems more than likely that William's wife, Elizabeth, came from Dartford, and one wonders if she was in fact also a Miss Williams — possibly an older sister of Sarah. Unfortunately the Dartford registers are illegible or non-existent for several years over this period, so that we have no record of either William Perfect's marriage or the baptism of little Elizabeth, which must be assumed to have taken place here.

The baptismal register for East Malling, however, clearly notes the baptism, on 19 October 1756, of 'Sarah, the daughter of William Perfect and Mrs Elizabeth his wife, by her grandfather the present vicar. Witness my hand, William Perfect'. This must mean that by then the young Perfect family had left Dartford and were in the Malling area. It had been arranged in the meantime that William would take over the practice of the elderly John Hicks, one of the doctors whom we find subscribing the licence of John Sisley, also of West Malling, in 1724, and it is possible that by October 1756 the Perfects were already installed in John Hicks' house, although definite proof of their having taken up residence there is not found until the next set of church rates, drawn up in April 1757. Here, Perfect's name is encountered for the first time in West Malling in place of that of Mr Hicks and misspelt, as Pafett, with the later insertion of an 'r' — a sure indication of a newcomer to a parish, with whose name the clerk or churchwarden who drew up the rating list was not familiar.

From late 1756, therefore, or early 1757, William Perfect, his wife Elizabeth, and their two little girls, Elizabeth and Sarah, were installed in West Malling, in the pleasant, double-fronted house, occupying a good position in the middle of the High Street, formerly inhabited by Mr Hicks. It was assessed, for rating purposes, at an annual rental of £8, a relatively modest sum, although slightly higher than those fixed on the houses either side of it. Henry Baker, on one side, was rated on a rental of £7, while William Lenham's house on the other side was assessed at only £5, although he paid another £1 for a stable, and possibly kept a small inn, which remains in use to this day, under the name of the Five-Pointed Star. Mr Hicks' house appears to have comprised an apothecary's shop as well, and it was from here that West Malling's new surgeon, apothecary and man-midwife, William Perfect, was now preparing and dispensing his medicines.

It is at this point however that it becomes imperative to consider the question of William Perfect's age. His date of birth is usually accepted as 1737, which would mean that he was only 20 when he began work as a doctor, and a mere 19 at the time of the birth of his *second* child. It would also mean that he had been apprenticed at the age of twelve, with the apprenticeship coming to an end when he was seventeen. Such a chronology seems rather unlikely. His later writing shows that he had profited from a classical education, and in spite of the fact that he was obviously a man of considerable gifts, it is hard to believe that his verse and prose could have shown such assurance and urbanity without the benefits conferred by a few more years of schooling. As the son of a clergyman, who, from William Perfect's later eulogies of him, appears to have prized learning as much as his son, he must have received as much education as possible, which would seem to imply that his father would have been unlikely to countenance an apprenticeship before the age of fifteen.

Nowhere is there definite proof of his age, but the dates in his early life make more sense if we posit 1734 as his year of birth, with an age of fifteen for his apprenticeship to William Everred in London in 1749. This would make him twenty when we find him in Dartford in 1754, apparently out of his apprenticeship, and twenty-two, perhaps nearly twenty-three, by the time of the birth of his second child, Sarah. Such a chronology seems somewhat more realistic, both for the son of a vicar, and for someone who always believed that the senses should be under the control of the reason.

As has been noted, the house which he occupied in West Malling, and where he lived for the greater part of his life, was a relatively modest one. When he began work as a doctor, William Perfect was far from wealthy, and his considerable achievements, in more than one field, seem to have been the result of hard work and dedication, aided by a very lively, sociable disposition. When he died in the summer of 1809, the *Gentleman's Magazine* carried the following obituary of him:

> At Malling, Kent, sincerely esteemed and lamented, William Perfect, MD, who, after having devoted a long life to the service of the most wretched of his fellow-beings, in the very skilful and humane exercise of his profession, may truly be said to have diminished the sum of human misery; while by the amiable and social qualities of his mind, and the generous and constant distribution of his property, he contributed in an equal degree, to the stock of sublunary happiness. His social and moral virtues will long be remembered by the Antient and Honorable Society of Free and Accepted Masons in that County; and the memory of their zealous and affectionate Grand Master will be long and ardently cherished; while the numerous dependants upon his bounty will do ample justice to the goodness of his heart, and acknowledge, with regret, that in him Humanity has lost a friend. As an author, he was well known, and not without merit.

As Samuel Johnson said, in lapidary inscriptions a man is not upon oath, and it seems reasonable to extend this to obituaries. However, all in all, as we shall see, that seems a very fair portrait of William Perfect.

Chapter 2

The Poor Parnassian Scribe

Very early, it would seem, William Perfect developed a taste for writing, and he was to say that he would almost sooner have become a writer than a doctor. In 1757 he had begun the first of nine folio manuscript books, which are now in the Masonic Museum and Library at Canterbury, labelling it 'Poeticae Compositiones Gulielmi Perfect 1757', and intending to copy into it all the verses he wrote — although he soon began to include prose articles, and copies of some of his correspondence received and sent.

The first volume in fact contains a number of verses and poems which are earlier in date than 1757, most of them in the pastoral mode, dealing with the loves of Colin and Delia (1756), or Colin and Clarissa (1755), or with the writer's ardent love for Florella, or Cleora, both written in 1757. Indeed, 'The Invitation', addressed to Cleora, is positively a 'Come into the Garden, Maud' (without the drama) written almost precisely a hundred years earlier (*Maud*, 1855):

> Come dear Cleora haste away
> Where cowslips gild the mead
> Where plumed songsters chirp alway
> And harmless lambkins feed.
>
> My gentle maid then come away
> Upon the plain be seen
> No longer dear Cleora stay
> But grace this smiling scene.

And similarly, another 'Invitation — an Ode to Phillis', written in 1755, rather more ardently:

> O come with all your heaven of charms
> And wing with joy my hours
> I'll gladly clasp you in my arms
> Amid our rural bowers.

If Florella, or Cleora, or Phillis was the Elizabeth who became his wife, we are not told. Most of the writing is on this semi-impersonal level, and it is only occasionally that we get a glimpse of the real people behind such drawing-room verse.

Verse which seems rather too light to merit much attention, perhaps? But it was very much to the taste of the day, and the reason that William Perfect, in 1757, proudly labelled a new manuscript book 'Poeticae Compositiones' was that he was already a published writer, and that a number of his poems had already appeared in a monthly journal known as *Martin's Magazine*. It is possible that the first poem in the MSS, 'A Song', addressed to a certain Daphne, and against which Perfect has noted, 'Inserted in *Martin's Magazine* for July 1755', was actually the first of his compositions to appear in print. Throughout 1756 and 1757 poems by him were appearing steadily in *Martin's*.

Gradually we get more serious things: translations or adaptations of Horace, for example, or paraphrases of Psalms. There is also 'Science, An Ode', against which Perfect noted: 'This piece trifling as it is I set the greater value by, as it was admired by my ever dear and much lamented father'. This appeared in *Martin's Magazine* for December 1756, and contains what is virtually the dedication of the writer to the cause of science:

> O then but Science Wisdom lend
> Let Fortune others sway,
> But deign to be your votary's friend:
> He'll gladly you obey.

'I don't mind about money'. But, as in the present age, life could be difficult without it. Money, and the property a man owned, with the status that conferred, made a lot of difference to what he was able to do at this time. Unlike the young Edward Hasted, the future historian of Kent, who was an almost exact contemporary, and who lived not far away, at Sutton-at-Hone, the young William Perfect could not dream of becoming a justice of the peace: for that, one required an estate worth at least £100 a year; nor did he have the qualification to become a turnpike trustee, that's to say, possessing lands or tenements of the clear yearly value of £50. Lesser positions would have been open to him as the owner of a house, positions such as a parish officer or a juryman at the sessions trials, but the career or profession which he had chosen did in fact excuse him from serving in these lower although essential posts. It is hardly surprising, therefore, that, denied a more active part in the local political scene, William Perfect should have found an outlet for his political views in his poetry. The poet can rise above considerations of position and wealth: he can address himself to the man in the street, or he can thunder at the secretary of state.

In 'Lines inscribed to the Honourable William Pitt', in June 1757 the whole country found itself addressed in an ode which began:

> Rise, Britons, rise, and meet Britannia's foe,

while in October of the same year Britannia was the recipient of the lines:

> Mourn, mourn, Britannia, and your loss deplore,
> For British courage can be found no more.

This was apparently written in the wake of the turmoil caused by Admiral John Byng's failure to relieve Minorca in 1756. Byng was condemned to death by a court martial in February 1757, but with a strong plea for mercy. The plea was overridden by George II, and Byng was shot in March of that year. William Pitt had supported the plea for mercy, a move which had caused a lot of wavering in his popularity, and in the following December Perfect sprang to Pitt's support with a very pleasant metaphor drawn from his own profession:

> I think 'tis unfit
> To doubt Mr P—tt,
> Whose laurels sure never can fade;
> He's not to be sold
> For title nor gold,
> Nor will he neglectfulness shade.
>
> Then what is this rout
> And turmoil about?
> Don't you know he's the nation's physician?
> Your boxes he'll fill
> With such sort of pill,
> As shall purge the late vile expedition.

Another squib, written in May 1758, and clearly on the subject of thief-takers and informers (the infamous Jonathan Wild had been hanged in 1725) aims in the direction of the blind justice of the peace, John Fielding, half-brother of the more well-known Henry:

> So Jonathan is still alive —
> Upon my word, it's odd
> That he should hanging thus survive
> And 'scape the ire of God.

The case is plain, the cause I see,
It undeceives my mind:
We now protect rank thievery,
And Justice, lo! is blind.

Perfect's satire, indeed, sometimes has the bite and wit of a Gillray
political cartoon, as in this 'New Song — Wrote at Maidstone, March 31st
1761' (on the occasion of the election of Rose Fuller and William Northey
as MPs for that town):

Let scandalous whispers no longer maintain
We sell our elections for profit or gain:
The rest of my life may I live in a den,
If the Freemen of Maidstone are not better men!
Derry down down down, derry down.

If ever we're bribed, it is only for sport:
A bribe is, you know, an amusement at Court;
In following Court fashions we'd nobody fright,
For the Freemen of Maidstone are much too polite.

Why ladies, for Hanger, your much beloved friend,
Abundance of voices the Poll did attend;
If we did not succeed, let us merit no blame,
For Fuller, you know, is a much fuller name.

Great sums were expended, so fame blazes wide —
Themselves for that fault must your candidates chide:
Had they stood but the chance without present or fee,
Why, we all to a man would have polled for all three!

Your hall shall be finished, says Northey at large.
Says Fuller, I'll give a magnificent barge!
Of your kindness, good sirs, let each Maidstone man sing:
God save our new Members, our freedom and King!

Now, now is the time we must rise to renown!
Hail, Aera that makes us a flourishing town!
While we boast of our men by election decreed,
May they never be fuller in word than in deed!
Derry down, etc.

This was printed in another paper, where Perfect had now become a
fairly regular contributor, *Mechell's Political Chronicle*. *Martin's Magazine*,

which had welcomed Phillis and Clarissa and their swains, was probably not the right home for these political and satirical effusions, and Perfect was now sending items to the *Westminster Journal*, as well as to *Mechell's Political*, or *Weekly*, *Chronicle*, as it seems also to have been called, while 'Mourn, mourn, Britannia' was inserted in the *Universal Magazine*, which also took several of his lighter efforts. It is now virtually impossible to track down most of these in print, but Perfect did in fact appear once or twice in that warhorse of eighteenth-century monthlies, the *Gentleman's Magazine*, which would have ensured his semi-anonymous immortality, if he had not himself published several volumes of his own verses. In September 1757, for example, over the signature G. P-f-t, the *Gentleman's Magazine* published his 'Beechen Shade', which concludes with the very Pope-ian lines:

> Let not the vain parades of wealth or show
> One wish of envy in my breast excite,
> But teach my heart this righteous truth to know:
> Enough for man — Whatever is, is right.

As well as political verse, there was also political prose. By the beginning of 1758, under the pseudonym of 'Probus', William Perfect was writing regularly to the editor, or, as he was frequently called, the author, of the *Westminster Journal*, who, like Sylvanus Urban of the *Gentleman's Magazine*, in real life Edward Cave, also had a pseudonym, and called himself Mr Simon Gentletouch. Perfect's epistles thunder in approved journalistic style, beginning with sentences such as: 'By the word Honour, Mr Gentletouch, I conceive is here meant a desire of fame or the applause of men directed to the ends of public felicity'; or, 'The irreligious principles of the present age induce me to expatiate on their gross and horrid consequences'.

Perfect also wrote as Probus to *Mechell's* Timothy Telltruth, another editorial pseudonym, and in this paper, between 1759 and 1761, he had a series of poems appearing under the general heading of 'The Artless Muse'.

Then for a while the journalism seems to have lapsed. Perfect wrote to his friend Daniel Shrimpton on 1 January 1762: 'I have for some time discontinued writing in public papers, as I have harboured a scheme to publish 2 vols. in octavo by subscription. When I am about to carry it into execution I will inform you' — and he was in fact to bring out his first volume of verse, *A Bavin of Bays*, in 1763. A single, fourteen-page poem, *An Elegy on a Storm which happened in West Kent on the 13th of August 1763*, was printed on its own in London in 1764. The advertisement for it, price 6d., in the *Kentish Post* in June 1764, also promised a larger work, price 2s., from the hand of the same author, W.P. *Calumny Dissected* would seem, from its title, to have been satirical or political in its content, but, if it did indeed come out, has vanished without trace. By early 1764, however, Perfect had again been persuaded to become a regular contributor to Redmayne's *Westminster Journal*, and poems from his pen, under the heading of 'Sparks of Pindar', were to appear throughout the year.

But 1764 was to see the even flow of William Perfect's life tragically disrupted. For nine or ten years there had been domestic bliss, marred only occasionally by a passing shadow. An ode, entitled 'Simple Morality', which had appeared in *A Bavin of Bays*, and which seems to describe the poet's own life, contains the following lines:

> Cleora, unassuming fair,
> Possesses all my breast,
> And sharing each domestic care
> Caressing is caressed.
>
> My little offspring blossom round
> And prattle as they play...

In 1763, when this appeared, the 'offspring' consisted not only of Elizabeth and Sarah, but also of William, born in 1758, Huntley Bigg (1760), George (1762) and Daniel Thomas, born in 1763. A shadow of some kind had certainly passed over the family in 1759, when Perfect, in his poem 'To resignation', had written that 'Distress instructs us, and is virtue's school'. Had there perhaps been a miscarriage or a still-birth that year? But tragedy came in June 1764, with the sudden and unexpected death of Perfect's wife, Elizabeth, possibly, again, as the result of a pregnancy. Like her husband, she was probably little more than thirty.

There is no direct mention of the event in the MSS, but six poems entitled 'Nights', or 'Night Thoughts', with an epigraph taken from Edward Young, and apologies for using his title, make Perfect's grief very explicit:

> O'er all my thorny festered breast supreme
> Sits sorrow president, and woeful fills
> The curule, which so late was pleasure's seat.
>
> (Night the First, 23 June 1764)

All nature slumbers, save the wretch like me,
Waked, torn and racked with sudden bursts of grief.
(Night the Second)

Thou, beauty's blossom, on fair Virtue's stem, ...
Torn from my bleeding breast (this breast of woe
Where midnight melancholy sits supreme
Beneath the cypress of my wakeful fate)
O my Octavia, blossom of my soul,
Blasted by death!
(Night the Third, 25 June 1764)

Elizabeth, as we learn from William Perfect's will, was buried at Dartford, which seems to confirm that town as the place she originally came from. The baby, Daniel Thomas, did not long outlive his mother, dying in October of that same year.

Such an abrupt end to his domestic happiness must have seemed almost unbelievable to the carefree poet, who had only had to walk beside the Medway, or wander in a friend's garden, to find inspiration for his muse. The poetical contributions to which he was committed for the *Westminster Journal* include the six 'Nights', and reflect his sombre mood for the rest of the year, while the overall title chosen for his contributions for the following year — 'Juvenilia, or Poems on trifling occasions by a Parnassian woodcutter' — may well indicate that he doubted whether verse would now flow from him as it had done before and that he might be obliged to fall back on earlier scraps, previously rejected. Nevertheless, there was an irrepressible, humorous side to him, which could smile even through grief — it was perhaps as well for his young family that this was so — and the contribution under the heading 'Sparks of Pindar' for 1 December 1764, 'Wrote a few minutes before dinner', already shows something of the old William Perfect peeping through:

Hunger, thou little peevish guest
Why am I thus by thee oppressed?
'Tis Nature's call — 'tis very true,
And to a poet nothing new.
But let me see what is to eat —
Why, faith, some wholesome-looking meat!
Pray, Cook, make haste, avaunt despair,
I'll eat away my hungry care! ...
Hark, dinner's ready — that's the call!
I fly! Muse, let your pencil fall!

Readers of the *Westminster Journal* for 25 January 1766 encountered a 'Prologue to the Poetical Botcher', and were informed that the first of this new series would appear on the following Saturday, and be regularly continued each week of the year, 'by Timothy Wildniss, esq', who mischievously added the two lines of Pope which had served as an epigraph to a popular volume of verse brought out in 1760 under the pseudonym 'J Copywell of Lincoln's Inn, esq.':

But when a Squire once owns the happy lines,
How the wit brightens, how the sense refines!

Nevertheless, as Perfect had sensed, regular inspiration was no longer so easy to come by. No doubt increasingly busy as a doctor, he was to welcome journalistic help from several sources. At least three of the items which appeared between January and March 1766 under the heading of 'The Poetical Botcher' are noted in the MSS as being by H Perfect, clearly a relative, but not otherwise identifiable.

Other friends and relatives also sometimes came to his aid. The Poetical Botcher No.23 was by Mr Skerrett, almost certainly the Thomas Gowland Skerrett who had married Perfect's sister Sarah in 1757 and who lived nearby in East Malling. In July 1766, during the course of a long letter to the Revd Thomas Austen, Perfect remarked:

You did promise to give me a few MSS for the *Westminster Journal*. They would be of infinite service to me. If you should think proper to transmit them to me, I will get them carefully published as from me signed T.A. ... If you have no objection I shall *Westminster Journal* your lines on Masonry.

No.24, accordingly, comprised the lines on freemasonry by Thomas Austen, to which Perfect had alluded in his letter, and Austen clearly sent Perfect a few more items, as he was thanked for them at the beginning of September: 'I am very much obliged to you for these sort of things, as they serve to help me out greatly in my hebdominal publication.'

Nevertheless, the Poetical Botcher seems to have disappeared from the scene before the year was out, and 1767 saw only an occasional contribution from Perfect in the *Westminster Journal*. However, on 1 January 1768 Perfect noted in his MS book:

Commenced writing for the *Westminster Journal* after dropping it for more than a twelvemonth. As follows:

To the Public. Simon Gentletouch desires to inform the public that having engaged four of the drollest geniuses to write for the *Westminster Journal* thro' the course of the present year, acquaints his readers in particular that their respective productions will appear weekly under the title of the Quadruple Alliance, or the Poets' Confederacy in favour of Simon Gentletouch, esq.

— which was a rather long-winded way of introducing very light verse! Who were the four poets? Perfect himself, of course, and the Revd Thomas Austen, undoubtedly. Thomas Skerrett may well have been the third — with 'H Perfect' perhaps making a fourth. But the Alliance seems to have fallen apart very quickly, and the *Westminster Journal* had to make the best of it minus its contributions from West Malling for the rest of the year. William Perfect seems to have had other things on his mind apart from his professional work and publications.

However, in January 1769 he announced to the Revd Thomas Austen, in one of his rhymed epistles, that the *Westminster Journal* had again applied to him for contributions, to be paid at the princely rate of three shillings a week:

> The Westminster Journal — by Gentletouch Sim —
> Solicits my aid — Shall it then have its whim?
> Three shillings a week — What, for verse and for prose?
> I must ever be seen then in thread-staring clothes!
> For this one year only to write shall I strive;
> The pay will scarce keep a church-mouse, Sir, alive.
> Three shillings a week! (Times grow worse and worse!)
> 'Twill never replenish (the) emaciated purse.

It is in this same letter that he announces to his friend both his second marriage — of which , he says, his friend will 'have heard — and have heard — and have heard' — and the birth of the first child of this marriage, another daughter. The letter contains the lovely line: 'The house is in odours with nutmeg and caudle' (caudle being a warm spiced sweet drink given to the sick and especially to women in childbed), but the letter is chiefly remarkable for the slightly defensive tone which Perfect adopts in describing his second wife — here called Lucinda, although in reality Henrietta. Henrietta seems to have been quite the opposite of Elizabeth the 'unassuming fair', with a quick tongue, and looks that it would be hard to praise:

> A girl, to be partial, I think more divine:
> Her tongue runs full fast, but her sense and good nature

Apologies make for this parrot-like prater.
Whoever described her possessed of the graces
Dealt not in the language of liking grimaces,
For the girl's well enough; — then as to her worth,
She's rich in a female, the first of her birth.

It has to be remembered, however, that William Perfect's second wife had to take on a family of five children, whose ages ranged between thirteen and six, and such a factor must have somewhat limited his choice, as well as rendering beauty an attribute of lesser importance. There is no further mention of Henrietta in the MSS, and she seems to have inspired no more verses, but there is no reason to suppose that she was not a perfectly acceptable wife and mother. She was to have three more children at, for the times, fairly long intervals: her first daughter, christened Folliott Augusta in January 1769, and perhaps named after Perfect's friend Folly Streeter, was followed by Lucy Dorothy Grenville in 1772, Thomas William Chamberlain in 1777, and Almeria Sarah Weller in 1779.

By then we are outside the period covered by the MS folios, which end in November 1773 — although Sydney Pope's article of 1939 on William Perfect noted that a further fifteen folio and quarto volumes of MSS written by him were sold in London in 1867. In 1771 Perfect appears to have had several poems published in the *St James' Chronicle*, while some 'Elegiac Lines Sacred to the Memory of an Affectionate Father' were published in the *Kentish Gazette* of Wednesday, 22 September 1773.

There is little doubt that he continued sending occasional poems and articles to the papers, using one of the numerous pseudonyms that he had adopted along the way: Probus, Pamelio, Chirurgicus, Hyperpoliticus, Lucius, and occasionally Pinxit Vivum, who supposedly wrote from Worcester.

It seems to have been generally known locally that he was a regular contributor to various papers, and the subjects of his wit and satire sometimes had little difficulty in identifying themselves. This seems to have been the case with a slightly scabrous description of a parish meeting which Perfect had written in 1759 for *Mechell's Chronicle*, and which began:

So! Convened to do something, a rum set of elves,
Who care much for their neighbours, but more for their selves,
A blacksmith, a barber, a cobbler, a priest,
As wise as the best, and of fools not the least;
With Hal, Dick and Roger, brave plough-jobbers all,

Who run to the alehouse at parish's call;
And Tipple a landlord, come out of the West,
When sober a blockhead, when drunk a bad guest;
With Skin'em, a miser, who ever is lost,
Except when to glut at the parish's cost...
Of hogs, geese and cows, they promiscuous prate
And drink, smoke and stink at a wonderful rate.

Whatever the pseudonym over which this appeared, the identity of its writer appears to have been guessed, for a month later another character sketch, entitled 'The Female Dun', had a new name appended to it: Perfect noted in his MS that 'to avoid the reflexions that some people have industriously spread of my writing "The Country Parish Meeting", it had been signed Pinxit Vivum, Worcester'.

Nevertheless, Perfect's identity must have been frequently guessed, and he did not normally go to very great lengths to disguise his authorship. The mask of the pseudonym was perhaps no more than the buskin of the actor: a convention of the theatre of journalism. In 1768, in what might well be called the Battle of the County Papers, when James Simmons, in Canterbury, was engaged in establishing the *Kentish Gazette* in competition with the *Kentish Weekly Post*, Perfect, as Probus, came down heavily in support of Simmons, writing a lampoon on the prime mover behind the *Kentish Weekly Post*, Thomas Smith, whom he accused of peddling inaccurate information and of being over-ambitious as well as avaricious, and concluding through the mouthpiece of Smith:

To obtain advertisements is all my delight,
And many I've taken to which I've no right;
My conscience is seared, and my face it is brass,
And the man that's more honest, I'd call him an ass.
For puffing designed, I'm beyond all compare:
I'm a Black-Smith by nature, deny it who dare.

Probus offered to provide facts to support his accusations, if the matter were taken any further, but Thomas Smith appears to have contented himself with an indignant expostulation that his late wife should have figured in the lampoon alongside himself.

The twenty years of journalism, poems, and a certain amount of correspondence contained in the MSS show us the man behind the doctor, from youth to middle age, a man of wide interests, but of a wholly consistent character. At one and the same time a son of the church and a son of the Enlightenment, he reproves atheists — as in 'A Word to the

Atheist' of 1754, and 'An Hymn to the Almighty upon the New Year' of 1755 – and pens 'An Ode to Science', disseminating medical advice in some 'Extempore Advice to a young gentleman concerning his conduct in Life':

> In eating my advice receive
> And moderation use,
> By rules of temperance learn to live
> And ne'er those rules abuse.
>
> In drinking e'er, my friend, refrain
> From what the health impairs
> Or may to madness drive the brain
> In Bacchanalian airs.

This good advice may well have been addressed to himself. He would only have been about 22 at the time – but it is perhaps worth noting that he had already had some thoughts about the causes of madness.

Politically, although schooled by his upbringing as a clergyman's son and by his medical training – and one should remember here the church's authorisation which he needed to practise as a doctor – to accept the status quo (and to echo Pope's line: Whatever is, is right), he held quite liberal views: he could inscribe an ode to the Society of Shipwrights of Chatham, 'who have, by voluntary contributions, erected a windmill for the grinding of corn in defiance of monopoly and extortion'; and toast John Wilkes, as follows:

> To Wilkes a long continued health:
> May he have share of peace and wealth!
> And may the year hight forty-five
> In British breasts be ever alive!
> And Number Forty-Five likewise
> Be ever honoured with the prize –
> A Laurel Crown – for this we pray
> Amen! – Huzza, Huzza, Huzza!

He was not, at the outset of his career, a rich man, and, as we have seen, did his best to ignore or despise wealth ('Let not the vain parades of wealth or show / One wish of envy in my breast excite'), but a lack of money could make life uncomfortable for a sensitive man. One of the Probus letters, sent to Timothy Telltruth's *Political Journal (Mechell's)* in 1758, had complained about servants of the well-to-do being allowed to solicit tips:

Scandal and ridicule have long been justly employed in reflecting upon our people of fortune and taste for suffering their servants to take tribute of those whom they kindly invite to their tables and perhaps honour with the appellation of friends ... Is it not shameful that a man of slender fortune cannot visit a nobleman, his friend and acquaintance, without paying the servants for their master's entertainment?

Both collections of verse which William Perfect brought out in the sixties, *A Bavin of Bays* and *The Laurel Wreath*, contain a number of poems which are to be found in the manuscript volumes. *A Bavin of Bays*, his first published collection of verse, was attributed only to 'a minor Poet'. It was published by subscription in 1763, and contains, among the subscribers, a number of locally well-known names, showing that Perfect was already widely known and highly regarded. The list of subscribers includes at least nine other doctors, and several reverend gentlemen. *The Laurel Wreath*, his second collection, which came out three years later, was slightly less coyly attributed to 'W.P.' This was again supported by a locally distinguished list of subscribers — as well as by John Wilkes, esq. — and the author says in his preface that it was 'by the particular encouragement of my friends and acquaintances that I became induced to suffer this collection of miscellaneous poems to appear in the world'.

Curiously, the two titles are very similar: the laurel, or bay, was used in ancient times to make honorary wreaths. A bavin is a bundle of kindling wood, so that a bavin of bays is a bundle of laurel twigs, perhaps ready for twisting into a wreath. The laurel, and its connotations, seems to have had a fascination for William Perfect. A letter written by him on the subject of honour and published in the *Westminster Journal* for 14 January 1758 laments:

How is the laurel wreath reduced from its pristine value! In short, Mr Gentletouch, it is no longer the glorious object of ambition, but is now so lightly looked upon as to be only estimated at the trifling value of the materials that compose it.

But this was perhaps merely an echo of a national preoccupation. Following the taking by storm of the strongly fortified island of Belle Isle by the Marines in 1761, during the course of the Seven Years War with France, they were granted the privilege of having a laurel wreath appear on their colours and appointments.

Half of the poems in *A Bavin of Bays* deal with the seasons and the months of the year; the rest are verses on a variety of topics, including a long poem on West Malling itself, and some humorous verse. The mixture of local colour and classical allusion is by no means unattractive, and William Perfect has a good ear and a good eye. 'January', for example, contains the following vignette, clear and sharp as the whistling it describes in the icy air:

> The plodding ploughmen, seized by piercing cold,
> Blow their numbed fingers or their arms infold,
> As through the fields they whistling stump their way,
> At morn or noon, or at the eve of day.

'August' paints a totally different scene, where 'paints' seems to be the operative sensual word, although no actual colour is named:

> The fruitful orchard now her tribute yields,
> And fair Pomona all her charms reveals;
> Each smiling scene allures the longing eyes,
> Pears press on pears, on apples, apples rise;
> Peaches on peaches swell in ruddy show,
> Nect'rines on nect'rines thro' the gardens glow,
> Figs over figs augment the gaudy view,
> And plums with plums contest for finest hue.

In 'September' the hop-pickers, coming down from London, are described with an unsentimental, but not unsympathetic, eye:

> They come in crowds, a wordy vulgar crew,
> Rush from Augusta, Kentish cares pursue,
> And native homes diminish on their view.
> Behold, how fast increase the rabble race,
> Some sue for pickers, some for binman's place;
> All have their wants and their diseases, too:
> Impoverished many, and half-starved a few,
> Till hopping 'gins; then those who starved before
> Are proud as princes, and are poor no more.

A Bavin of Bays also tells us a little more about William Perfect himself. 'April', for example, reveals him to be a keen fisherman:

> Though humble, yet the angler's part be mine,
> Armed with the trowel or with the strong-spun line ...
> Well stored with worms or artificial paste
> Brooks to their sources shall by me be traced,

> While I with various baits am well supplied
> I'll cheat the rivers of their finny pride.

The 'finny' deaths no doubt provided the Perfect family with some excellent fish dishes. Perfect had no objection to the legitimate pursuit of food, but he was totally against hunting for mere sport. 'August' contains a quite impassioned plea on the subject:

> Heart-aching thought! shall man delight to spill
> Offenceless blood, and for diversion kill?
> While savage beasts, if not by hunger pressed
> Unstained by blood would in the forests rest?
> Ye wanton tyrants, who delight in blood,
> Is joy in pain? is glee at anguish good?

Nevertheless, exceptions could be made: we find Perfect himself taking out a licence to shoot game in 1787. Perhaps he restricted his shooting only to those items intended for his family's (and/or his patients') consumption!

Like *A Bavin of Bays*, *The Laurel Wreath* contains a number of poems on local themes. The first one, entitled 'Barham Place, the Seat of Sir Philip Boteler, Baronet' is virtually a dedication of the book to Sir Philip, whose house at Teston overlooked the Medway. This river, the principal one in Kent, flows through both books almost like a unifying theme, and was obviously much loved by William Perfect. In *A Bavin of Bays* he had written of 'Old Medway's fertile banks', and 'barge-bent Medway'; here we have, perhaps a little more stiffly, 'glassy Medway's serpentine tide'.

The Laurel Wreath also has several attractive elegies, among them one on his father, and another entitled 'An Elegy to the Memory of a deceased friend', who appears to have been Fraser Honywood. Here again, as in the poem 'August', with its description of the hop-pickers, we find a recognition of social concerns, on the part of both poet and subject:

> Possessed of blessings, willing to impart,
> His ear was open to the orphan's prayer;
> Misfortune found a passage to his heart,
> With others' sufferings ever prone to share.

> Ask who to helpless infancy alone?
> Or who to feeble age assistance lent?
> Who soothed the weeping widow's melting moan?
> The stranger cheered, with painful wandering spent?

Charity of this kind, from having been derided as patriarchal, seems now to have been totally extinguished in our culture: although a more even distribution of wealth is undoubtedly a sequel to be desired, and which Perfect's friend, who is praised for his generosity of spirit as well as of his hand, might have recognised. Perfect himself seems to have felt indebted to him for recognition:

> Who fed the hungry poor from bounty's hand,
> With eye impartial saw low merit rise,
> And, though in rags, approved what wit had planned,
> Foremost to vindicate the muses' prize?

The Laurel Wreath also has its humour, particularly in the tour de force, 'A Shop Bill Versified', which Perfect seems to have written for his West Malling friend, the grocer Joseph Wilkins:

> I J–h W–s, of the grocery calling,
> And facing the Swan, in little Town Malling,
> Sell pattens and clogs, penny histories and ballads,
> Train, lamp, barber's, shoe, oil, with finer for salads;
> Fine ink and ink-stands, black and red sealing-wax,
> Knives, scissors, red herrings, and shoemaker's tacks;

And the ninety lines, and several hundred-odd items — a social study in themselves — end goodhumouredly with what must have been anathema to a trained doctor, a list of patent medicines:

> And, what's more important, I deal in some slops:
> The Elixir of Daffy, and Bateman's famed drops;
> By the patentee's licence, I give them to sale,
> With the Cordial of Godfrey, which never will fail;
> Elixir of Radcliffe, British Oil, and Scotch pills,
> And Hooper's Specific, for feminine ills.

'A poor Parnassian scribe', a phrase in which William Perfect referred to himself on more than one occasion, may also have made reference to a joke between him and his friends. In 1760 there appeared *The Shrubs of Parnassus*, published by J. Newbery, and attributed to J. Copywell, of Lincoln's Inn, esq., containing, as the title-page stated, 'a variety of poetical essays, moral and comic'. In subject matter this verse was not unlike that attempted by Perfect: the occasional love-song, topographical poems, elegies on the deaths of friends or the famous (*The Shrubs of*

Parnassus contains one on the death of Admiral Byng), and addresses to humble objects. Both Copywell (or W. Woty, as he is now thought to be) and Perfect were much indebted to Pope, and *The Shrubs of Parnassus* has for epigraph the two lines of Pope which Perfect was also later to borrow.

Only a year later there was a follow-up to *The Shrubs of Parnassus* in *The Scrubs of Parnassus*, brought out by another publisher, J. Williams, and mentioned in the *Gentleman's Magazine*, but now seemingly lost. Although the title makes it sound satirical, it was probably also an attempt to catch the attention of the same market which had found the 1760 book to its taste: *The Shrubs of Parnassus* had had a surprisingly long list of subscribers, who included among their number Samuel Johnson, Tobias Smollett, John Wilkes, David Garrick, and Samuel Derrick, the Master of Ceremonies at Bath, as well as numerous surgeons. It was to have at least one more sequel, in which William Perfect himself was to be involved.

It seems to have been some time after Perfect's own volumes of poetry had appeared, that is to say, probably during the 1770s, that some of his verses, which he had originally noted in the MSS as never having been published, were, according to a later note, given to Folly Streeter for his *Weeds of Parnassus*, a book of which there now seems to be no trace. It was perhaps not quite so barrel-scraping as the name might seem to imply, including such items as 'An extempore description of a sudden tempest at sea', which Perfect had noted as having been written by the seaside at Rye in July 1756, and a poem of 1755 entitled 'Happiness, in imitation of the first ode of Horace's third book'.

Folly Streeter would appear to have lived in Chatham, and to have been in all probability the F. Streeter who published in 1778 a small book called *Hampton Court*, containing some poems and a farce in two acts, which he had printed by T. Fisher, the Rochester bookseller. Streeter does not seem to have been a doctor, but he clearly shared William Perfect's interests in three things: poetry, medicine, and the stage. The farce, *The Physical Metamorphosis*, is preceded by a note to the public, in which Streeter says:

> Some friends having desired the Quack Doctor's speech to be delivered on the public stage, with the necessary apparatus to set it off: it could not, with any degree of propriety, be introduced, without the addition of some scenes, to give it a shadow of probability.

And Streeter goes on to explain that his play exposes all the various schemes and cheats practised on 'the credulous poor' by mountebanks pretending to be doctors. The play appears to have been performed with Mr Streeter taking the demanding role of Dr Diureticdiacalonchrocus-linimentemsapernatem, whose mountebank speech is some two and a half pages long, and very possibly with William Perfect in another part. There is every likelihood that Perfect contributed the book's short 'epitaph', which is noted as 'Wrote by a Friend', and which seems to bear the Perfect stamp:

> What man of wisdom would write verses?
> When he must still lie at the mercies
> Of every scrawling critic band
> By whom his writings must be scanned!
> This is the poet's blest condition:
> A second Popish inquisition;
> For when the trial's undergone,
> The odds a thousand is to one,
> That in the Critics' corner's crammed
> The writer, and the writing's — damned!

The lighthearted tone of this is altogether characteristic of Perfect's attitude to his writing and its reception. Poetry was for him one of the joys of life — but only one. There were many more, including friendship, recorded for us in the correspondence, and often bringing with it the transient but remembered pleasures of a day's outing or a visit, when the doctor would be gaily mounted on 'My horse, in person rather scant, / Between Buceph and Rozinant'.

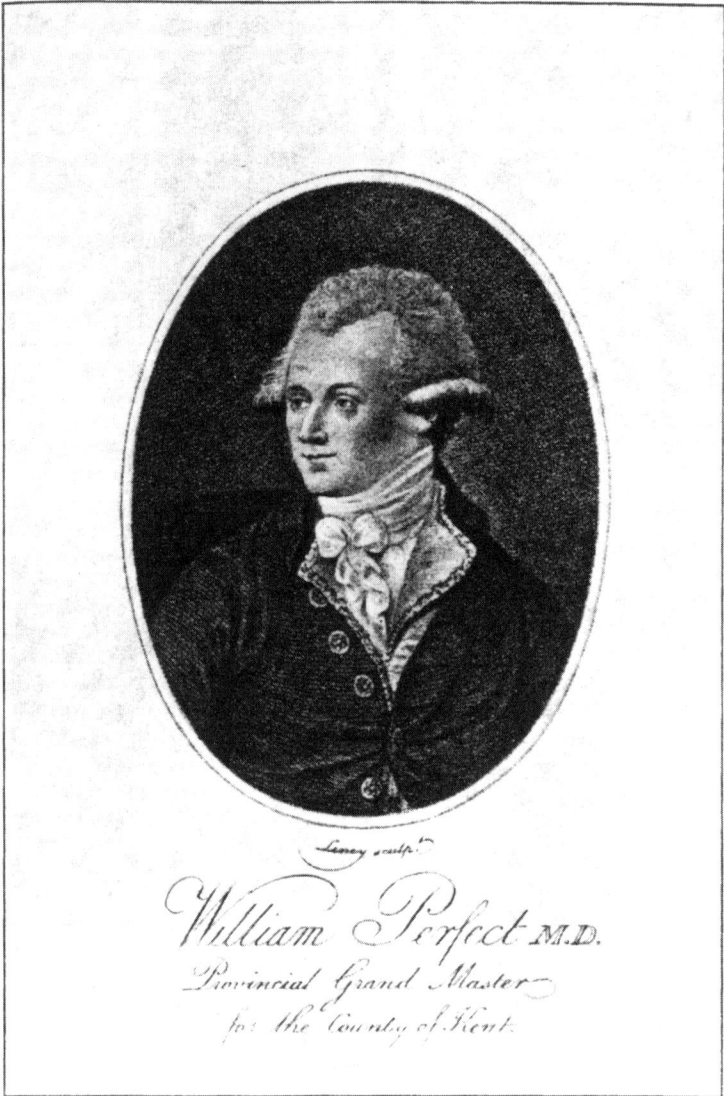

William Perfect M.D.
Provincial Grand Master
for the County of Kent.

William Perfect aged about 40.

Chapter 3

Friends and Freemasonry

As a doctor, William Perfect had an immediate entree into the houses of the well-to-do in the area — of whom there was quite a number, particularly in the swathe of parishes lying to the west of the Medway, between Aylesford and West Peckham — and his wit and education clearly brought him the friendship of several of them, among whom may perhaps be named the Earl of Aylesford, the Earl of Westmoreland (at Mereworth), Sir Philip Boteler (at Teston) and, nearer home, at West Malling, Fraser Honywood.

Perfect seems in fact always to have had friends on various social levels, several of them, like himself, keen lovers of poetry and literature. His clerical friend, the Revd Thomas Austen, vicar of Allhallows in the Hundred of Hoo and a minor canon of Rochester cathedral, has already been mentioned. In 1766, by the hand of Mr Streeter, Perfect sent Austen a book, *The Beauties of Poetry Displayed*, so that Austen might add to his own poetry commonplace book from it. Thomas Austen seems to have offered to provide additional poetic copy for the *Westminster Journal* in 1766 — 'When you want materials for the *Westminster Journal* you must let me know and I'll do my best at all times' — and, as we have seen, was probably one of those who formed the Quadruple Alliance in 1768. The correspondence between Perfect and Austen was not invariably on a high-flown level, and could even be scabrous. William Perfect had a good sense of humour, and in any case, as a doctor, must have been well acquainted with the foibles and frailties of mankind. In one of his letters to Austen he quotes Swift, speaking scathingly of people who are 'dead to pleasure themselves and the blasters of it in other people — mere dogs in a manger'. It was perhaps a disappointment to Perfect that his friend disapproved of his acting. The stage clearly had great appeal for him, and he seems to have contrived to take a part on various occasions, whether it was to oblige a friend, or to help out a travelling company. In August 1757, for example, he both wrote and spoke the prologue for a performance of *Cato* which took place at the Golden Lion at Brompton, and in 1766 was to tell the Reverend Canon that his admonitions came too late:

Let me not incur your displeasure when I ingeniously confess to have offended very grossly against the friendly dictates you gave me in point of stage-playing. I was sincerely obliged to you for your advice, and should very seriously have declined all those things, (if) had I not previously promised young Jarrett of Chatham that I would play Chamont in *The Orphan*, and when your admonition reached me I had studied the part so thoroughly, and was so well versed in it, that I should not greatly have hesitated to have been seen in it on any public stage.

As to the reflexions of the world, the longer I live the more I perceive, and with pain I perceive, them to be the sole productions of malice, envy, ignorance or ill-nature, and, to deal freely with my friend, am quite grown indifferent to what defamation, from her snaky throne, may throw upon the light-built fabric of my reputation. I have most egregiously suffered by report, and without any cause at all, and shall never attempt by grimace to make the world think better of me than I deserve.

Perfect seems to have taken the same part again in 1773, when a company of players was at the Assembly Rooms in West Malling, as well as writing and speaking a prologue which began as follows:

The muse, unpractised in the rules of art
To melt by tragic tale the feeling heart,
No doubt has scruples, both of shame and fear,
To venture unprepared an object here.
If some should think myself I now degrade,
Let 'em remember, 'playing's not my trade';
Or, if it were, such scorn I could endure,
To please myself, or to relieve the poor.
'Twas Charity alone that made me dare
Usurp the tragic walk, and turn the player.

Another activity in which he indulged, and about which we learn from a letter to Austen, was the occasional game of cricket. Austen, mistaking Erasmus's parish, which had in fact been Aldington, had told him that the Dutchman had been rector of Addington, and Perfect replied:

I shall now venerate the village accordingly, insomuch that, belonging to a club there frequented by the principal inhabitants, I shall most likely take a trip with them to Chatham on Tuesday to engage in the obstreperous game of cricket, not to oblige myself, observe, but purely for the sake of the famous and learned Erasmus being once Rector of a place where I have now the honour to be a member of a beer club.

Another corresponding friend was Daniel Shrimpton, of Islington, who may have been the son of a City of London doctor, William Shrimpton. Perfect wrote to him in October 1760, sending greetings to 'the Islingtonians', and proposing a monthly correspondence 'which I love to support with those whom cruel space denies my seeing so often as I could wish'. This seems to have been mainly on literary subjects: earlier in the same letter Perfect had said:

> Poetry you know was always my favourite amusement. The study I must acknowledge still pleases me, but as my avocations increase am obliged to pay my devoirs to the nine ladies much seldomer than my natural bent inclines me to do.

And in a postscript the doctor and poet requests Shrimpton to buy for him Orrery's *Life of Swift*, and Rasch's *Observations on Surgery and Midwifery*.

There were also local friends and acquaintances, the merchants and tradesmen of West Malling, some of whom formed a club which met at the Bear, and about the members of which, including himself, Perfect sent Shrimpton some rhymed 'caricatures':

> A dull set of mortals at evening repair,
> To smoke a dull pipe at the sign of the Bear;
> In number two dozen, their names, trades, and so,
> Shall follow in order: observe them below.

Very fairly, Perfect describes himself first, among this 'dull set of mortals'. Then comes West Malling's other doctor, Thomas Rowley:

> The tribe pharmaceutic my muse must prefer,
> So the second is Fracture, you know him, good sir,
> Not a Compound, but Simple, he enters and stands,
> Then rubs his rough knuckles to whiten his hands.

And Perfect is equally uncomplimentary about his conversation: 'No one understands him, so some think him wise'. But the tour de force is perhaps the sketch he draws of Fowler, a cooper:

> Some sign-painter sure drew the third on the list,
> His name, why it is, Sir, Vociferous Twist!

A bracer of barrels, a cooper by trade,
By the Lord of the Manor our Clamourer made.
Of his oven-like mouth I but little shall say,
But I must of his chin, for it hangs in my way.
It contains a good acre, nay, some will say more,
And one saucy fellow protests near a score!
E'er I finish this figure, one note I must make:
His voice is designed for to keep us awake.
With mechanical wisdom, though mean in condition,
Our Cryer sometimes will commence politician.
He well understands all the schemes of our foes,
And says, 'As how, rat it, he very well knows
Where the Hisland of Molta did use for to be,
But what argues that, why it stands in the sea!
As to what they're about up at London, Lord rat 'em,
Pitt cannot be Pitt now he's made Earl of Chat'em!'
For threepence he swills down a gallon or near
(From this bright silver tankard) of fourpenny beer.
This hogful replenished, he wakes us no more,
But bears home his chin for a sounding-board snore.

There were clearly many other friends in William Perfect's life, of whom we know little or nothing. There was certainly someone called Bigg, as there was probably someone called Huntley, after whom his son Huntley Bigg must have been named — Bigg or Biggie is mentioned in one or two of the letters, — while the Chamberlain in the name of his son Thomas, and the Grenville and the Weller, in the names of his two youngest daughters, Lucy and Almeria, are probably also the names of friends who may have been called on to act as godparents.

The abrupt end to the MSS in 1773, with the conclusion of Volume 9, means that the detail which they provide is lacking for the last thirty-six years of William Perfect's life. However, another facet of this many-sided man was his attachment to freemasonry, and this provides us with some records for his last two decades. It seems to have been in about 1765, fairly soon after the death of his first wife, Elizabeth, that William Perfect became interested in freemasonry. The subject was frequently raised in letters to his Rochester friend, the Revd Thomas Austen, during 1766, and around that time he noted down in his MSS a 'List of all the Lodges in England down to 1765 with their number and date of establishment'. This begins with nine set up in 1721, including ones at the Queen's Arms, St Paul's Churchyard, at the Horn, Westminster, at the Sun and Punchbowl, High Holborn, and at the Crown and Bells, Chancery Lane, and gives the first one in Kent, number ten on the list, as that established at the Globe in Chatham in 1723. Perfect also copied out a Latin motto for a lodge, which he translated, and whose precepts seem to accord quite well with what we are able to know of his own character: 'Know thyself, place thy trust in God, pray, avoid show, content thyself with little', and it ends: 'learning the art of living well and that of dying'. Given the date at which these entries in the MSS were made, it seems possible to say that William Perfect turned to freemasonry for consolation on the death of his wife.

Although he is assumed to have become a freemason in 1765, it is not known to which lodge he originally belonged. However, he is thought to have become a member of the True and Faithful Lodge in Dartford in 1775, and to have been instrumental, in 1787, in the transfer of this lodge to West Malling. Freemasonry would seem to have had a great appeal for William Perfect, both for its moral tenets and also for the memorised ritual which provided the framework for its meetings, and which had in it something akin to the theatre, which he had always loved.

It was to be in freemasonry that he achieved his greatest social distinctions. In 1787, by now an MD, and entitled to be addressed as Dr Perfect, he was promoted to be Provincial Grand Orator, an office which no longer exists, but which must have suited his histrionic talents. Seven years later, in 1794, on account of the severe illness of the then Provincial Grand Master, Colonel Jacob Sawbridge, Dr William Perfect was recommended for the office in his place, and on 18 May 1795, by a patent from the Prince of Wales, Grand Master of the Free and Accepted Masons in England, was appointed Provincial Grand Master for the County of Kent. His Provincial Grand Chaplain, appointed in 1795, was the Reverend Jethro Inwood, who later dedicated to Perfect a volume of masonic sermons.

As Provincial Grand Master William Perfect had power to make masons, and to constitute and regulate lodges. Several new lodges were indeed warranted in his time, although none of them seems to have been very long lived. They included the Jacob's Lodge at Ramsgate (1798), the Lodge of Reason at Ashford (1799), and the Perfect Lodge, warranted in 1796, and instituted at Woolwich by Matthew Garland, who in 1797 followed in Perfect's steps by becoming Provincial Grand Orator.

The naming of a lodge after the county's Grand Master was perhaps a vindication by the freemasonry of what outsiders may have seen as somewhat high-handed behaviour when, in 1792, Perfect's own lodge, the True and Faithful, had circularised all the lodges of England warning them against accepting as a freemason one Thomas Smith, 'of the neighbourhood of Maidstone, dealer in rags', who had been expelled from the West Malling lodge as 'a violator of decency, and all those laws by which men of honour and reputation bind themselves, abandoned to the grossest immoralities, a dishonour to Masonry, and unworthy the name of man'. In case he should try to get accepted under another name, there followed a lively physical description of Smith:

> a man of middle age, swarthy complexion — sometimes wears a dark queue wig, at other times his own hair tied behind — about five feet six inches in height — has lost some of his fore teeth by fighting — generally wears a blue coat and makes a shabby appearance — has a jeering manner of speaking, with a forced smile upon his face — loud and low in conversation, and some time ago followed the occupation of tinker.

Thomas Smith brought a case against William Perfect to recover damages for libel, and was awarded £50 by the jury. However, it seems curious that the only other known case in which Perfect was prepared to attack a man's character also involved a Thomas Smith, and it seems unlikely that he would have risked his reputation without grounds.

Among other duties as Provincial Grand Master William Perfect was called on to preside at the annual meeting of the Provincial Grand Lodge, held in various towns in the county where it was hosted by the local lodge. This took place in 1797 at the Sun Tavern in Chatham, in 1798 at Ramsgate, in 1799 at Maidstone, and in 1800 at Michener's Hotel in Margate. There was some particularly serious business to attend to this year, since, in the political climate engendered by the French Revolution, freemasonry had fallen under the suspicion of being a seditious society, a suspicion which no doubt all Provincial Grand Lodges strove to allay. The Provincial Grand Lodge of Kent, considering that 'As a veil of secrecy conceals the transactions of our meetings, our fellow subjects have no assurance that there may not be in our association a tendency injurious to their interests,' felt impelled to reveal that it was one of their fundamental rules never to discuss politics. Another disturbing recent event had been the attack on the life of George III by James Hadfield, later found insane, and committed to Bedlam: the Grand Lodge of Kent, through the mouth of their Grand Master, made a 'humble and dutiful address to the King, congratulating him on his late providential escape from the daring hand of a sanguinary assassin'; although one cannot help feeling that the innocent prayer 'That Providence may long continue to defeat every daring and dark attempt, even of insanity itself, that is aimed at his sacred person' approached, albeit unconsciously, too near to the King's own personal tragedy to offer the solace that was intended.

Part II: THE DOCTOR

Chapter 4

Smallpox and Obstetrics

We can say with some certainty that William Perfect began his medical career in West Malling in 1757. He was fully qualified by his apprenticeship to another surgeon to call himself 'surgeon, apothecary and man-midwife', and, as we have seen, there are clear signs that he had made good use of his time as an apprentice, attending lectures on midwifery given by Dr Colin Mackenzie, and very probably accompanying him round the wards of a hospital as well.

Midwifery had only recently established itself as part of the routine practice of a doctor. Before about 1730 female midwives had virtually monopolised the profession, certainly outside London, and to a large extent in London itself. Until then, the role of the doctor as man-midwife had extended only to surgical intervention in emergencies, so that he had tended to be lacking in any very extensive experience of normal childbirth. Around 1730, however, occurred what is known as the obstetric revolution, when doctors began to take a much deeper interest in midwifery per se, and William Perfect's studies in this area, and the book which he subsequently published, show that he was at the forefront of this medical interest. He was still liable to be called on to help out in an emergency — midwives were undoubtedly cheaper than doctors and their services remained popular — but he was quite prepared to undertake standard deliveries. The man-midwife, by the end of the eighteenth century, was no longer a novelty, although he was never to outnumber the female midwife.

The surgeon was the general practitioner of the eighteenth century, dealing not only with broken and dislocated bones, and all diseases and injuries which required manual operation, but all external diseases, those of the skin and of the eye, dressing wounds and ulcers, opening abcesses, and removing teeth. The treatment of venereal disease also came within his purview. The apothecary prepared his own drugs, and usually had a shop, from which he sold them to the public. Apothecaries also formed a separate profession, and in newspapers of the time one not infrequently comes across advertisements for an apothecary's shop, either for sale or to be let. In November 1758, for example, the *Kentish Post* was advertising 'A Compleat Apothecary's Shop, with all its Tinctures and Utensils, with some Drugs', for sale at Strood, while 'A good-accustom'd Apothecary's shop, with the furniture, etc', was to be let at Yalding.

William Perfect's training equipped him in all these fields, and he must, in some wise, have spread word around that he was now installed at West Malling, as its new surgeon, apothecary and man-midwife. He himself does not seem to have placed an advertisement in the paper to this effect, but other Kentish doctors, on setting up practice, were keener to advertise, frequently offering free services over a limited period. The four following gentlemen all placed an advertisement in the *Kentish Post* between April and July 1757:

> Charles Fagg, surgeon, apothecary and man-midwife, in Ashford. Having been instructed in the art of midwifery, under William Smellie MD in London, gives this public notice that he will attend all those who shall apply to him for the space of one year, gratis.

In May, John Twyman, setting up as a surgeon and man-midwife in Thanet, was giving notice that 'he will attend all such women as may want assistance in any cases of midwifery within 5 miles of Birchington for the space of six months, gratis', while in the same month readers learnt that:

> William Francis, surgeon, apothecary and man-midwife (from St Thomas's Hospital) ... has opened an apothecary shop in St Margaret's near Hawk's Lane, Canterbury. And will be ready to give his attendance on all persons that desire it.

Ashford saw some competition to Charles Fagg, in the person of William Coleman, surgeon, apothecary and man-midwife, who, 'having taken the shop lately Mr Adcock's at Ashford, deceas'd', notified the public that he 'will continue selling druggs, chymicals and galenicals, at the lowest price, as usual'.

Although William Perfect is chiefly remembered in Kent today as a doctor for the insane, he spent many years practising as a general surgeon, with all the varieties of case and circumstance which that entailed. From a letter copied into his MS book in 1765, for example, we know that he attended Maidstone gaol, where he deplored the custom of denying a decent interment to the corpses of hanged men, stripped and flung into a common burial pit, and he seems to have retained his interest in conditions in the gaol, for in the winter of 1784 his name appeared in the

Kentish Gazette as one of the gentlemen willing to receive donations for the relief of the prisoners there 'in their present great distress'. Towards the end of his life he may have been consulted almost exclusively on matters relating to insanity, but before that he had become something of a specialist in two other areas, namely, inoculation against smallpox, and midwifery.

Inoculation for smallpox, although practised in Turkey and possibly neighbouring areas much earlier, was only introduced into this country in 1721. It was taken up cautiously, and frequently condemned for spreading infection by church and parish authorities alike. A breakthrough came in the late 1750s, when a Suffolk doctor, Robert Sutton, improved on the method by which it was performed, developing what became known in the hands of his sons as the Suttonian method, which passed on the infection more lightly and safely. One of the sons, Daniel Sutton, moved to Ingatestone in Essex, and having carried out a great many inoculations there, including, apparently, some general ones in parishes threatened with epidemics, wrote to the authorities at Maidstone, offering to perform a general inoculation there which would contain the ravages of the disease.

Sutton's offer seems to have been made partly with a view to enlarging his smallpox practice into Kent. Doctors had undoubtedly performed the operation in the county before this, most notably, perhaps, Daniel Dobel at Cranbrook, but the general inoculation at Maidstone in the summer of 1766 both publicised and popularised it, and from 1767 on the county paper began to be filled with advertisements from doctors offering inoculation by the new method. William Perfect was one of these. His long insertion in the *Kentish Post* of 21 January 1767 announced that he was now inoculating 'according to the new practice which thousands have happily experienced to be the most safe and successful method'.

If he did not himself witness any of the inoculations carried out by Daniel Sutton — and the Suttons were very secretive about their method — Perfect was obviously fascinated by them, and it was probably not difficult to find someone who had been inoculated who was articulate enough to describe the method in detail. To a doctor's eye, the benefits offered by successful large-scale inoculations were huge: they could mean a virtual wiping-out of this devastating disease which, if it did not kill, always disfigured. Perfect's jubilant verses, entitled 'The Inoculator Triumphant, or the Smallpox totally Vanquished', were inserted in the *Westminster Journal* for 30 August 1766, and must have been written very shortly after the successful incursion into Maidstone by the East Anglian inoculator. The speaker is clearly a doctor: part Sutton, who may already have had several thousand inoculations to his credit (although hardly millions!) and part Perfect, eager to jump into the fray and 'outdo them all'!

> Attend to my theme, every rank and degree!
> Ye lasses so lovely, come listen to me!
> Oh, how you'll caress me on knowing my skill,
> Who love in the cause for to flourish my quill!
>
> All marks on your bosoms or scars on your face
> My art shall prevent your dear forms to disgrace,
> My practice enjoins you no diet severe
> And is equally good at all times of the year.
>
> The gross and scorbutic, the hectic and aged
> To inoculate safely I must say I've engaged.
> Fame's trumpet may sound it all thoro' the nation:
> I cure the smallpox, and without inflammation.
>
> By my potent art that disease is defied
> I've cured near a million when one has not died;
> I've so conquered Pandora, and let the world know
> When I give the word she no farther can go.
>
> The Doctor may shake his unfortunate head,
> And say with a sneer, 'He can raise from the dead!'
> At my miracles rare let the Faculty brawl:
> My practice shall show that I outdo them all!

An Aylesford doctor, Humphrey Porter, had been advertising his services in this field as early as December 1766, and in the following February, less than a month after Perfect's first advertisement had appeared, the two doctors notified the public that they had now entered into a partnership for the purposes of inoculation, with a house fitted up at Aylesford for the accommodation of patients. The partnership seems to have been successful, for it was soon extended, not only further into Kent — where Porter and Perfect undertook a general inoculation at Elham, and opened a house for the reception of patients at Wye — but also much further afield.

Success clearly bred envy, for in June 1768 the two doctors were obliged to place the following insertion in the county paper:

> Whereas it has been industriously propagated by ill-natured preju-
> dice ... that Messrs Porter and Perfect, surgeons, of Aylesford and
> Town Malling, in Kent, have lost patients by inoculation both in

this county and other parts of England ...[*a reward of 200 guineas is offered to anyone proving that they*] ever lost a single patient by inoculation; that any one has had the smallpox a second time ... Such persons who chuse it may be taken in and genteelly accommodated, during the short space of inoculation, in their dwelling houses at Aylesford or Malling. ... The poor of parishes are undertaken and attended upon easy terms.

The nasty, and clearly untrue, rumour was obviously scotched, and the two doctors' reputations remained unsullied. At the end of October, 1768, they were reporting that they had established partnerships with doctors in other parts of the country. Quite how this worked is unclear. It almost goes without saying, however, that at this time any method proposed by one doctor would have been modified or improved by another, rather in the way cooks improve on each others' recipes, and the method of inoculation offered by Porter and Perfect, while almost certainly based on the Sutton method, was almost as certainly a variant of it. It quite possibly included dietary instructions, to be followed beforehand in order to ensure that the patient, on inoculation, was in as healthy a state as possible, and medicines to assist in recovery afterwards. The instructions, and the requisite medicines, would have been distributed to the participating doctors who must have been visited from time to time for the purpose of renewing their supplies and collecting the fees due. Perfect seems to have had hopes of rivalling the Suttons in numbers inoculated, but by 1769, although there is some evidence that this was not the last big journey he undertook, he had begun to feel that the return was too meagre for the outlay in time and money. This is expressed in one of his rhymed letters to the Revd Thomas Austen, that of January 1769 in which he announces the birth of little Folliott Augusta. Mentioning that he has been ill, Perfect continues:

I now am recovered, intending to roam
Once more for some hundreds of miles from my home.
This journey my last, for to settle accounts,
And to see to what sum all our labour amounts.
Contest then who will for advantage o'er Sutton,
Forbidding in regimen, beer, beef and mutton,
So small now's the fee for this wholesome invention,
'Tis even too poor for a poet to mention;
Besides, when my partners call to divide
But little is left me to pay for my ride;

And when I cry, Sirs, see, here's my disbursement!
They'll cry that they never saw money much worse spent!
So I will no longer contend for their pelf
But strive where I can to collect for myself.

That he still continued as a smallpox doctor, however, is shown by his advertisement of February 1772 in the *Kentish Gazette*, in which the public were notified that for the purposes of inoculation,

> Mr Perfect, surgeon, Town Malling, continues to take patients into his house, from four guineas to one. In the course of several years' practice he has inoculated many thousands, without the loss of a single patient.

1766 was also the year in which William Perfect took on an apprentice. Pury Samuel Caister, the son of a yeoman of Foots Cray, signed an indenture as was customary to the effect that he of his own free will, and by and with the consent, good liking and approbation of his father, Henry Caister, yeoman, 'put himself apprentice to William Perfect of West Malling ... Surgeon and Apothecary to learn his art'. The indenture was dated 14 August 1766, the apprenticeship being for seven years from that date. The premium paid for this was the extraordinarily low one of ten guineas. Was Perfect doing the boy's family a favour by asking so little? Medical apprenticeships at this time usually paid a premium ranging between £50 and £100; William Perfect himself, or rather his father, had paid a premium of £30 in 1749. It is true that Pury's family undertook to provide clothing and to see to his washing, but this is unlikely by itself to have accounted for the very nominal sum asked by Perfect. From his well-formed signature, Pury Caister would seem to have belonged to the category of older apprentices, and it may be that Perfect felt his intelligence and probable usefulness should outweigh mere pecuniary considerations.

However, the apprenticeship did not work out satisfactorily. On 2 January 1770 Pury informed his master by letter that he intended to apply to Quarter Sessions (as was necessary) to have the apprenticeship discharged, giving as his reasons that Perfect had not had 'sufficient business and practice to teach and instruct me in the art and mystery of a surgeon and apothecary', and also that he had not 'in many instances been used by you as an apprentice ought to be'. The indenture was accordingly dissolved by the signatures of four magistrates at the January Quarter Sessions at Maidstone. Perhaps we need not take Pury Caister's complaints too seriously. It was necessary to furnish reasons for this legal step to be taken, and it is just as likely that Caister had come to feel that he was in the wrong profession, and wanted to do something else. He did not seek an apprenticeship elsewhere and never became a doctor.

For some years after that two of Perfect's sons, William and George, who both became surgeons, may have served their father in a similar capacity although they were not formally apprenticed to him. In the very first issue of the *Maidstone Journal*, in January 1786, Perfect is to be found advertising for an apprentice to a surgeon 'in extensive business in the western part of this county' (as well as for a cook) but we do not know what the outcome of this was.

It is hardly surprising that, as someone who enjoyed writing, William Perfect should have committed to paper a number of the medical cases he encountered. There are several instances of the publication of single cases which he wrote up. As early as February 1758 he had a description of a case of catalepsy inserted in the *Gentleman's Magazine*, over the pseudonym Chirurgicus. In 1763 Volume I of the *Medical Museum*, a collection of medical pieces, contained a short anatomical paper by him on 'Appearances upon opening the body of a woman who died ... after eating a large quantity of cucumbers'. He also contributed 'An attempt to improve medical prognostication' to Volume III of the same publication, a paper which was noticed by the *Medical Register* on its first appearance in 1779. But it is for the books which he published himself that he is best known. His first medical book, *Methods of Cure in Some Particular Cases of Insanity*, came out in 1778, and his second, *Cases in Midwifery*, in two volumes between 1781 and 1783.

The material in the book on midwifery is on the whole earlier in date than that in *Methods of Cure*. The very first case in volume one is dated 19 May 1761, and towards the end of volume two there is a case which occurred on 21 September 1781, so the complete work covers twenty years of obstetric cases of particular difficulty or interest, encountered by a country doctor or man-midwife in the second half of the eighteenth century. Of particular interest for the social historian is the background to each case, which frequently indicates the social level of the women whom Perfect was called on to assist, as well as their activities during pregnancy.

Many of the women encountered in Perfect's pages seem to have paid little attention to the fact that they were pregnant. At least one of the women overstrained herself while harvesting. Another got into difficulties by 'hastily stepping over a stile'. Another 'fell from her horse'. Yet another, M.H., 'a woman of the sanguineous temperament ... was suddenly taken with convulsions and fell into labour ... after sitting up a whole night to dance'. Convulsions, or fits, are mentioned surprisingly frequently in connection with labour, as are fainting fits; and frights or shocks cause miscarriages on a number of occasions: the poor woman who 'hastily stepped over a stile' was recovering from this mishap, during her fourth pregnancy, when she had the misfortune to hear of a fire in the neighbourhood, the shock of which sent her into fainting fits, from which she subsequently died. One gains the impression, from looking through William Perfect's cases, of a womanhood which was physically robust but mentally somewhat delicate.

Physically robust, of course, if they had been well fed and nurtured from birth. With the poorer people this was often not so. One of the cases, dating from 1768, concerns a poor woman of 33, whose pelvis had been distorted by rickets in her childhood — quite a frequent occurrence, says Perfect. This woman had been in labour for three days and nights, with a midwife to assist her, when Perfect was sent for by order of a parish officer. Although complimentary on other occasions about midwives, he is here very critical of the 'ungentle' handling the poor woman had been given by hers. There are a number of occasions, among the cases recounted, when Perfect mentions being sent for by order of an overseer, or other parish officer, to help a woman in distress, not just in West Malling, but in several parishes in the area, including Leybourne, East Malling and Ryarsh. This shows the welfare system of the eighteenth century at work: the poor were not simply left to die, not were they at the mercy of quacks: when it was absolutely necessary, the best medical attention was called in. On 2 January 1780 Perfect was 'desired to visit Ann Phinnis, a pauper, belonging to the parish of East Malling, who had been in labour 3 days and nights, and was attended by two midwives'. This was another dangerous case, but William Perfect's skill enabled both mother and child to survive the ordeal.

Case CII gives us details about a gipsy confinement:

> In the night of the 3rd of September, 1772, I was sent for in great haste to the assistance of a gipsy woman, who was in labour in a barn, about 2 miles distant from this town; she was a strong, healthy woman, and had borne three children, with all of whom, she informed me, she had been delivered by herself, without any kind of assistance; had always had easy labours, and soon got well.

This time, having gone a month past the time when she reckoned her baby was due, she is found to be carrying twins, both of whom, with Perfect's care, are born alive.

The woman was so well on the sixth day, that I met her walking in the high road, with one child at her breast, and the other tied to her back. In about a fortnight after this one of the children died, and she brought the other to me, that I might look at its eyes, as she said something covered them like a skin, and the child had not been seen since it was born; upon examination I discovered a very thin filmy coat.

Perfect was able to perform the minor operation which removed this, and concludes: 'and I presume, that the operation fully answered the design, as I neither saw or heard any thing of the matter afterwards'.

One of the cases, which had been communicated to Dr Colin Mackenzie by letter, was that of Eleanor Emmerson, another travelling woman, to whose aid Perfect was called in 1762 by a neighbour who found her in labour in a barn.

She ... was exceedingly weak and low for want of nourishment, of which she had tasted no kind for the last twelve hours ... As she was wretchedly poor, and in a most low and dejected condition, my first step was to procure her some warm caudle and a few necessaries, which the exigency of her case seemed to require at the hand of humanity.

Eleanor Emmerson was also carrying twins, both of whom, with Perfect's care, were born alive.

In spite of this specialisation, however, William Perfect retained a lively interest in all aspects of his profession. Indeed, in 1769, no doubt remembering how useful he had found the lectures he had attended as an apprentice, he was himself offering a general course of medical lectures, advertising in the *Kentish Gazette* in September:

William Perfect, Surgeon, with the assistance of a gentleman of the first eminence in medicine and anatomy, has prepared and is ready to deliver a private course of lectures upon anatomy, the theory, principles, and modern practice of physic and surgery. He humbly presumes his design will be found of particular utility to the younger practitioners, and tend to compensate for the want of opportunity in such who have not attended lectures of this kind in London.

Chapter 5

The Mad-Doctor

Perfect's book on midwifery went into three editions. Volume I had borne a dedication to Samuel Foart Simmons MD, who may well have been Kentish — he is found as a subscriber to several books on Kent which were coming out around this time, including William Gostling's *Walk in and about the City of Canterbury*, of 1774. From the language of the dedication one does not gain the impression that they were close friends, but they were obviously acquainted, a fact which is of interest, as Simmons was also in the process of becoming a mad-doctor. He became physician to St Luke's Hospital for Lunaticks, and, although not given much recognition in this respect, he was also a physician to George III, appointed as such in 1803. In 1812, two years after George III's final mental breakdown had begun, a parliamentary committee examined the king's physicians 'Touching the state of his Majesty's health' for the last time, and Simmons was one of those called upon to give evidence.

It is unlikely that Perfect had studied under Simmons, since Simmons was younger than he was, but in his Preface to *Methods of Cure*, Perfect mentions his indebtedness to several other eighteenth century medical writers on lunacy, including the well known Dr William Battie. There is clear evidence that he read widely, and although he was to develop his own 'methods of cure', he certainly did not ignore the findings of others; in his Preface he was to express his hope that others, in turn, would profit from the dissemination of his own knowledge and experience.

The treatment which he meted out seems to have varied with each case, and he proceeeded experimentally, making sure that there were no adverse reactions to whatever it was that he prescribed. In the manner of the times, he was a great believer in bleeding — known variously as phlebotomy or venaesection — and in blisters, but he also made a considerable use of drugs in the treatment of nervous disorders. Many of these were of course drugs prepared by himself. He found an acid elixir of vitriol particularly helpful, as well as Boerhaave's strengthening chalybeate tincture, which he prepared from the following recipe:

> Take of filings of steel one ounce
> of very sharp distilled vinegar ten ounces

of sugar three ounces
Boil them 26 hours in a tall phial, and when filtrated, preserve the
infusion in a glass vessel.

Given the good effects obtained with this chalybeate tincture by
Perfect, in common no doubt with many other doctors, we can perhaps
understand a little better the eighteenth century's appreciation of natural
chalybeate water, in spas up and down the country. Another substance
which he found efficacious was camphor.

Perfect seems to have had a concept of holistic treatment: not
infrequently, patients who came under his care had their diet controlled
— although this could mean encouraging greater liberality — and the
'warm pediluvium', a comforting footbath, was often prescribed. By the
time of his death he seems to have been making some use of electric shock
treatment, although there is no mention of it in his book, which deals
with cases up to 1781. In his will, Perfect bequeathed to his son George,
who was to continue his 'business and profession of insanity', not only
'all my books on medical, surgical and obstetric subjects of every description', but also 'my electrical machine'. He was not a pioneer in this: from
at least 1756 John Wesley, who was a doctor before he was a preacher, was
finding electric treatment beneficial for nervous cases of all kinds, and
others took it up also.

William Perfect seems to have been interested in — and perhaps
horrified by — madness from quite an early age. In a poem of 1756 he
advises a friend (or possibly himself) to refrain from excesses in drinking
which 'may to madness drive the brain' (and he was to treat a number of
alcoholics); and some correspondence of 1761 shows that he already had
an active medical interest in restoring people to their senses — if not
actually recovering them when others would have given them up for dead.
In November 1761 his friend Sally Williams of Dartford, was writing to
him:

> You sent Robinson home almost his own man again, and he
> continues to mend in his looks very much. But I don't think he has
> quite got his speech yet: if he talks for a little while one may perceive
> an hesitation which he did not use to have, but one can't expect to
> have him firmly established yet. It is next to a wonder that he is not
> in the number of the dead, and I hope he is sensible of the mercy
> received.

In his book, *Methods of Cure*, Perfect does not mention any cases
anterior to 1770 — at least, he does not give any earlier dates, although the

cases are mostly undated. By then, however, he was already known as a specialist in the treatment of insanity, as we can tell from the very first case, which begins: 'A gentleman, aged fifty-eight, was, in the beginning of January, 1770, put under my care for insanity.'

It seems safe to assume from this and from the other evidence that we have that Perfect had been building up his expertise, and treating cases of lunacy, for some years, taking into his home, when required, not only patients for inoculation, but those whose mental disorder required supervised treatment.

Not all madhouses were as carefully conducted as William Perfect's, but even the most scrupulous madhouse keeper was not always able to prevent its use for unscrupulous ends. Scandals concerning madhouses began to stir the public conscience in the middle of the 18th century, and the result, somewhat delayed, was the passing in 1774 of the first Act of Parliament 'for regulating Madhouses'. Until then, it had been possible for anyone to run a private house for the reception of the insane, with no safeguards against the ill-treatment of those held in them, or against the incarceration of people whom others, usually relatives, might find it more convenient to have out of the way.

In 1763 a parliamentary committee had been appointed to 'inquire into the state of the private madhouses in this kingdom'. It was probably in support of this action that the *Gentleman's Magazine* noted the following case, which had been reported in the *Historical Chronicle* for December 1763:

> A bill of indictment was found by the grand jury at Westminster against the master and servants of a certain mad-house, for unjustly detaining a young gentleman 13 months, and using him cruelly. It is said his pretended friends met him on board an Indiaman, and took him, with his effects, which were considerable, into a coach, and instead of taking him home, as they pretended, carried him to this mad-house, where, though in his perfect senses, he was confined in a strait-waistcoat, tied down 17 nights and days, denied the use of pen, ink, and paper, and otherwise used so ill that he spit blood; but at length, by getting some Morella cherries and a tooth pick, he found means to let his case be known to an acquaintance, who soon after procured his liberty.

The committee actually examined several complainants who had been confined in madhouses, some of them in Mr (later Sir) Jonathan Miles's madhouse at Hoxton, which had been established in 1695, and which was to continue well into the next century, as well as eminent physicians who specialised in lunacy, Dr Battie and Dr Monroe, both of whom were very definitely of the opinion that madhouses required regulating.

However, it was not until another eleven years had gone by that the necessary Act was passed, and even then it was fairly limited in its scope. Under this Act, it was not permitted to keep more than one lunatic in a house without a licence, and no one was to be admitted as a lunatic without an order in writing, under the hand of a physician, surgeon or apothecary. Licences, outside London, were to be granted by Quarter Sessions, and the Keeper of the madhouse had to enter into a recognizance of £100 with two sureties of £50 that he would 'be of good behaviour'. The Keeper also had to notify the College of Physicians of the admission of a patient within 14 days and his premises had to be inspected once a year by two visiting justices and a physician.

The Act was only concerned with the liberty and welfare of those admitted to private madhouses as private patients: it did not cover insane paupers, of whom quite a large number were boarded in private mad-houses at the expense of their parishes, nor those who might be found in general hospitals, workhouses, or poorhouses. One can probably assume, however, that public institutions had little interest in confining persons unless they were demonstrably raving or dangerous. By 1774 William Perfect's interest in caring for, but more particularly in curing, the insane, was well developed, and he had already established a reputation for this. We find him, accordingly, entered in the Quarter Sessions minutes each year as having entered into the necessary recognizance of £100, with Leonard Miller, a yeoman, of Ryarsh, initially accepting responsibility for the two sureties of £50, and entering into a further recognizance of £100. The licence itself would appear to have cost Perfect £15 a year.

It was by no means a large establishment. William Perfect's licence allowed him 'to keep lunatics not exceeding the number of ten', but we should not be misled into thinking that he always had this number of mental patients. He certainly had more than one, or he would not have needed a licence, but until shortly before 1780 they were, in the manner of the time, and like the patients coming to him for inoculation, accepted into his own home, where the space had to be shared with his growing family: his tenth and final child, Almeria, was to be born in 1779. By 1780, however, he was able to buy additional premises in the town: a small house assessed at the annual rental of £2. This would have been fitted up with suitable apartments for his patients, but again, may have housed no more than four or five.

Charging a fee was perhaps a delicate matter. In an advertisement which he placed in the *Kentish Gazette* in May 1774, Perfect mentioned that 'A consideration equal to the patient's case and circumstances will be expected'. The 'consideration' probably lay somewhere between two and five guineas a week. Apart from boarding his patients Perfect also had to pay those who attended them, including at least one muscular assistant, to help in the control of the more violent cases. Interestingly, the West Malling parish registers note the burial, in December 1786, of one John Clow, who is described as 'black servant to Mr Perfect', and it seems possible that John Clow may have filled this role in the Perfect asylum.

A few years after the passing of the Act for the Regulation of Madhouses, Perfect felt the need to make his services more widely known, and he brought out an eight-page *Address to the Public*. In this he praised the wisdom of the legislature in passing the 1774 Act, although from the description which he gives of the treatment meted out to the insane in many madhouses, such an Act had not come before time. Too many men and women, says Perfect, instead of receiving lenity and compassion, and gentle and humane treatment, have been kept in gloomy cells of torment and misery, where savage and barbarous keepers

> have punished with the hand of relentless severity their cries and lamentations, which evinced the sense of all their woes and injuries, as the clamorous ravings of madness and phrenzy, and often anticipated by these nefarious acts of implacable rigour and sordid knavery, the very evils which they should have endeavoured to redress and prevent.

He, William Perfect, on the contrary, has been able 'to lay down a probable plan of cure for insane and lunatic persons, the epileptic, hypochondriac, hysteric, nervous and such as labour under species of fits, which daily exhibit a dreadful scene of all the miseries "human flesh is heir to"'. And he continues:

> Without boasting of superior skill and judgment in these cases, I have treated them with such tenderness, attention, and success, as to meet with the approbation of the impartial practitioners of physic, whose great abilities must for ever silence illiberal censure, and invidious detraction — I am happy to make here a public acknowledgement for their kind and generous assistance, and their spontaneous recommendations.

Perfect emphasises the advantages to his establishment of his having been regularly trained in surgery and pharmacy, and of the detached and commodious apartments which have been fitted up for his patients. Nor were the poor, by reason of their poverty, necessarily excluded from treatment:

> Parish Officers and persons whose circumstances will not allow them to treat upon terms fully adequate to Mr Perfect's more enlarged plan, will find him disposed to receive patients for a limited time, on conditions consistent with his benevolence and humanity.

Alternatively, if it was medicines which their case required:

> That the friendless and indigent might not be excluded from the benefit of them, those who labour under any of these infirmities of body or mind, in bringing Mr Perfect a certificate signed by the minister of their parishes signifying their helpless and impoverished circumstances shall henceforth receive one course of his medicines gratis.

The *Address* recommended Perfect's book, *Methods of Cure*, which was available for 2s.6d. from Fisher in Rochester, as well as from two London booksellers, Dodsley in Pall Mall, and Conant in Fleet Street, and it concluded with a Latin quotation from Van Swieten, 'Ad sanitatem animi morborum mansuetudo, humanitas, patienta, plurimum conferunt' (Gentleness, humanity and patience towards the sick contribute much to soundness of mind).

If William Perfect's pamphlet seems somewhat overblown, even for the times, it could well be that he was expecting to see more madhouses established in the wake of the 1774 Act, some of which, if they were in London or North Kent, could be in competition with his own – and the eighteenth-century doctor was always alert to the possibility of competition. In the event, however, his was to remain the only one in Kent for many years, and his reputation grew accordingly. In 1776 Charles Seymour, in his rather brief *Survey of the County of Kent*, devoted the best part of a page to William Perfect and his madhouse:

> Mr Perfect, a skilful and experienced surgeon ... has fitted up divers convenient apartments for the reception of all persons insane, or immersed in the desponding abyss of melancholy. They are attended at his house with the affection of a parent, and the abilities of a man, who has, from study and observation, reduced into a practical science the method of restoring the most vital and most extrensic

madness to cool sense and rational judgment. This gentleman, actuated by a noble principle of universal benevolence, and a tender concern for the mental infirmities of his fellow creatures, has so far succeeded in the arduous task of curing dementated individuals as to deserve a singular favour and countenance from the legislature.

In the following cases, taken mainly from *Methods of Cure*, we can see some of the people who came to occupy William Perfect's 'divers convenient apartments'. The cases also serve to illustrate the treatments of the day meted out by other doctors as well as by Perfect.

CASE IV

A lady in the 37th year of her age, of a delicate constitution, in lying-in of her second child, and about a month after her delivery, was seized with a shivering fit, succeeded by a fever, delirium, inflammation of the eyes, and watching. [*She is somewhat better after three weeks, but is then upset by something in her husband's conduct.*] She became anxious, irresolute, incoherently talkative, turbulent, and so mischievous, that her attendants were obliged to confine her; raving, foaming at the mouth, involuntary laughter, or loud lamentations ensued; from a pleasing, open, chearful countenance, her face was contracted to a rigidly emaciated and truly maniacal appearance; and, from a decent and delicate choice of words, her expressions bordered upon blasphemy, or vented the rankest obscenity. The general methods had been referred to, under the direction and care of a most eminent physician, by whose advice she had been four times bled, within the space of three months; blisters had been prescribed for the occiput, back, and legs; a seton had been fixt in her neck; to lenient purges cathartics had succeeded; the gums, and fetid anti-hysterics, had been administered in abundance; vomits often prescribed, and cold-bathing not omitted. All painful applications, and every method hitherto used, had rather aggravated than lessened her complaint; and in a state of insanity little short of raving, she was committed to my care in May 1773; she had then a blister upon her back, and an issue in her arm; but as no good effect had ever accrued from muscular irritation, they were both suffered to dry up, and in a few days there was no discharge from either.

I lodged her in a quiet, retired, darkened room, gave her magnesia, to occasionally relax the bowels; and, for the heat and quickness of pulse, two spoonsful of a neutral mixture every 5 or 6 hours, with an addition in the evening of a few drops of the paregoric elixir. In ten days the spasms abated, the febrile heats were allayed — the pulse, from near a hundred, was, at times, reduced to below 80; when a decoction of the bark, with nitre, was made use of. [*The intervals at which this medicine is given are gradually increased, from a few hours to a day or two, then to a week, and from a week to two weeks.*]

During the continuance of this course, I suffered no one to visit or converse with her but myself and one female attendant, the relations and acquaintance being strictly enjoined from the first not to come near her. By means of the above practice, retirement and a regimen properly adapted to her case, in November of the same year, I had the happiness to restore this lady to her worthy partner and family, and the chearful reception of a large circle of genteel acquaintance, who had experienced many anxious feelings on her deplorable situation.

In the next case, psychotherapy comes into play.

CASE XIV

A lady, about the age of 30, by long-continued grief and distress of mind, for which she had in vain sought relief from change of place, company and climate, was in November 1776 attacked with an hysteric fit, in which I was called to assist her. [*She proves difficult to treat: Perfect tried to 'soothe her nights with opiates', but to these she had 'so constitutional an antipathy', that he had to discontinue them. Other treatments were tried, including an emetic, which brought on a three-hour fit. Eventually Perfect found she slept well after 3 spoonsful of camphorated julep.*]

The narcotic efficacy of the camphor, in some few instances, I had experienced before; but in this case it was most particularly so. A decoction of orange-peels with Boerhaave's most excellent strengthening chalybeate, was prescribed to her twice a day; and, with much solicitation, she was prevailed on to be more liberal in her diet, and chearful in her conversation; which, in a few weeks, removed the solicitude of her mind, and braced the habit to its pristine tone.

The following case deals with a gentleman aged 45 who suffered from a severe depression:

CASE III

Mr S.G. about forty-five years of age, after having for some years been subject to acute rheumatic pains, and the internal haemorrhoids, on a sudden, without any apparent cause, became low-spirited, dull, and melancholy, insomuch, that he was unable to follow his business as usual; he was frequently watchful, timorous, mistrustful, and despondent, and more than once, if he had not been providentially prevented, would have put an end to his existence; he was first attacked in the beginning of September 1772, and had then tried the advice of an apothecary in the place where he lived. In November I received a message to visit him, and found him seated in his customary attitude, his head reclining on his arm, and his eyes riveted to the ground, as if lost in profound thought; I tried by several methods to rouse his attention, but to no purpose, and asked him several questions, but received no reply at all ... When I took him into my house, he had, I think, the most incurious aspect which I ever beheld, and was so nearly approached to a degree of confirmed idiotism, that a servant was obliged to dress, undress, feed, and assist him in the common offices of nature. After a few days, I bled him, to the quantity of six ounces; the complexion of the blood proved the vessels to be loaded with a superabundant quantity of humours, which clogged and loaded the circulation so as to render depletion highly necessary. I prohibited his wonted freedom of diet, and confined him to a more slender and cooling one; he was often carried into the air, and took daily, in a bason of water-gruel, two drachms of soluble tartar. The pulse was greatly relieved, and softened by the first bleeding; by the second, (at the distance of fourteen days) the effect was more promising; and, by a strict perseverance in the antiphlogistic plan, with repeated bleedings and a proper degree of exercise, the patient became susceptible to the dictates of propriety, sensible to the functions of nature, and entirely recovered his right senses and understanding. The regimen now was gradually enlarged; and for some time after taking a decoction of valerian and the bark, to invigorate the system, he left me hearty and well in the March following, having come to me in November only.

And Perfect noted at the end of this case:

Since this cure I have had three melancholics much relieved by phlebotomy ... and a few months since I had a case of the kind from Marden, where venaesection had universally been prohibited by every gentleman of the faculty who had seen her; and yet this patient recovered by repeated bleedings only.

The full title of the first edition of Perfect's book was *Methods of Cure in Some Particular Cases of Insanity: the Epilepsy, Hypochondriacal Affection, Hysteric Passion, and Nervous Disorders*, and he does in fact group his cases under these heads. Some of the cases would clearly not be considered as insanity today: alcoholism, for instance, of which he gives two or three examples, and the girl who suffered from fits brought on by worms. His methods varied enormously, and depended greatly on close observation of his patients. He never seems to have proceeded in any course to which they objected, but he was open to the merits of a number of treatments practised at the time. Thus, although in the case of the lady of 37 who was brought to him after the birth of her second child he could see that blistering was quite wrong, he found it helpful in the case of a gentleman of 58, the subject of Case I.

Two forms of 'insanity' perhaps seem to us particularly connected with the eighteenth century, and William Perfect gives examples of both. The first of these concerns a case of hypochondria or melancholia about which Perfect was first consulted in December 1770. The person in question was a young man aged 22, of Carey Street, London, who had been disappointed in a marriage treaty, and who from a cheerful disposition, became

> sad, dull and pensive, destitute of his wonted resolution, with almost a total loss of appetite, sleep, and spirits, and fond of solitude; for some week together he scarcely spoke a word, and from a florid complexion became pale and wan.

Up to this point it seems no more than the typical melancholy projected by Romantic literature, 'alone and palely loitering' with Keats, or weeping over a lake with Lamartine. But the remainder of Perfect's description of this case shows that it could be a much more distressing illness than that:

> In about three months after this melancholy dejection took place, he was seized with a drivelling, which continued four or five days, and during which time his speech was facilitated, his appetite mended, and he enjoyed a partial return of his wonted vivacity; but no sooner did this discharge leave him than he reverted to his former gloomy and dejected state. A physician of eminence had in vain been consulted, and the ptyalism periodically returned with every full moon, brought with it its exhilarating and left its distressing effects. In this state he continued for the space of eight months, when he was entrusted to my management and care on the

15th day of January 1771.

Briefly, Perfect treated him with mercury to cause sputation, and carried him over the next two new moons; he bled him, advised purging draughts at the change of every full moon; and the young man, fully recovered, left William Perfect's house at the beginning of the following May.

Another type of mental disorder treated by Perfect, which was very much symptomatic of the age, but which we might not have expected to go as far as insanity, developed out of religious enthusiasm. As the son of a church of England clergyman, and also as someone who believed in the primacy of reason, William Perfect was wholly against such excesses, as we can see in the case of Mrs E.H., 'of a florid complexion, full habit, and about the age of 48', who 'had for some time past paid so strict an attention to a favourite system of religion, which like a kind of epidemic contagion, has long spread its baneful influence through so many ranks of people, to the excitement of the most daring outrages and wildest extravagancies, that at length she became insane'. Perfect continues:

> And if it be true, that instances of insanity are at this day more numerous in this kingdom, than they were at any former period, we have great reason not only to attribute the cause to the universal diffusion of wealth and luxury through almost every part of the island, but also to support the opinion, that so humiliating a degradation of our reasoning faculties owes much of its accession to the absurd tenets and ill-founded notions of an epidemic enthusiasm, whose type is absurd and gloomy notions of God and religion, derived from vulgar prejudices, which excites the attention of weak understandings to points of religion, which they contemplate without comprehending, to the entire subversion of their rational faculties.

Mrs E.H. appears to have been one of those who were excited to 'wildest extravagancies', but in less than two months Perfect had reduced his patient to a state of abstemiousness, and her wild antics and religious fervour had begun to abate; at the end of eight months religious enthusiasms were entirely annihilated; and at the end of twelve months, 'seeming consistent and rational, she returned to her family, who carefully guarded against her relapse by a total prohibition of the zealous devotees to whom she owed the first impressions of her disorder'.

A similar, although quieter, case was dealt with by the patient being allowed to see no books of a religious tendency and being forbidden the use of a testament, which 'she had been suffered to have in her possession', while the servant was ordered 'not to answer any interrogations she might propose upon pious matters, or even to speak to her thereon'. Fresh air and walks were called on to assist in the case of this cure, which took no more than seven weeks.

Methods of Cure in Some Particular Cases of Insanity, from which most of these examples have been taken, came out in 1778. A second edition appeared around 1783 and a third, revised, edition, under the title *Select Cases in the Different Species of Insanity,* in 1787. This was dedicated to John Coakley Lettsom, MD, FRS and AS, who was director of the City of London Lying-in Hospital from 1785 to 1815, and whose permission to dedicate Perfect described as 'a proof of private friendship, and a record of your own feelings, whenever humanity can be exercised or displayed'. In all, the book went into seven editions, the last of which came out in 1809, the year of Perfect's death. Hunter and Macalpine say of it that it was

> the first collection of psychiatric case material and even if it added nothing new to the progress of the art, it is a record of the kind of patients met with, the observations considered worth making and the variety of treatments administered.

There is perhaps a question-mark over the reasons for the initial appearance of the book. It could well have been intended, originally, as a super-compendious advertisement: 'I, William Perfect of West Malling, can cure the following cases'. There was heavy medical advertising at the time, frequently with descriptions of cases cured, and it is possible to see William Perfect's book, certainly in its first edition, as merely a collection of such cases in book form. Nevertheless, it was a novel thing to do, and, particularly in its revised form of 1787, *Select Cases,* the book served, as Hunter and Macalpine say, to 'form the basis of Perfect's reputation as a mad-doctor both among his contemporaries and in the history of psychiatry'.

Additional details about some of the inmates are to be found in the minutes of West Kent Quarter Sessions. As well as recording William Perfect's licence each year — at least between 1775 and 1805 — the Quarter Sessions archive also contains a few reports which were made by the visiting justices and physician to his madhouse, as had been stipulated by the Act. These usually took the form of a statement that they had visited the house kept for the reception of lunatics by William Perfect 'and after examination heard of no complaint but what might reasonably be imputed to the unhappy circumstances of the cases, and found the house in good order and fit for the purpose intended'. It must have been difficult for the visiting justices to know quite what to expect. However, it was not impossible to differentiate betwen cases, and there were two occasions when the justices and visiting physician made representations about patients confined in Perfect's institution.

The first of these occurred in October 1787, when Henry Hawley and Dr Thomas Milner reported:

> That Job Tripp confined in the said house as a lunatic (and put in there at the instance of his younger brother William Tripp) upon his own representation of his case as well as upon the best enquiry we could make did not appear to us to be a lunatic or to be a proper object to be confined in the said house.
>
> That the said Henry Hawley by and with the consent of the said Dr Milner did two days after to wit on the 7th day of August wait upon the said William Tripp in London and did represent to him the situation of his brother, his earnest desire to be released and our opinion concerning the impropriety and injustice of his continuing to be confined as a lunatic.
>
> That on Tuesday last the 25th day of September the said Job Tripp was conveyed from Malling in the balloon coach by Dr Perfect with the intention as is alleged by said William Tripp to carry him to London and to release him from his confinement. That when they had proceeded 5 miles to Wrotham the said Job Tripp was arrested at the suit of William Fowler of the Castle Inn in Maidstone for a debt of £23.10s. contracted some years ago and was directly conveyed to Maidstone Gaol where he now is.

All in all, a splendid instance of pure (and verifiable) eighteenth century farce!

The case of Sally Gaitskell, noted down in the minute book at the West Kent Quarter Sessions for Michaelmas 1803, was more serious:

> Report of visits by Sir Henry Hawley, Bart., and Francis Smith, Doctor of Physic, to house kept by Doctor Perfect at Malling, licenced to receive insane persons, 18th December 1802 and 19th September 1803, with particular reference to the case of Sally Gaitskell, detained against her will.
>
> Dr Perfect says, he cannot put her at liberty, without the permission of her friends who put her under his care. And here we must beg leave to submit, how far Doctor Perfect is strictly justifi-

able in detaining this patient against her will, at the request of her relations, or on any representation whatsoever, when he, the Keeper and Physician of the house, is of opinion that the patient is of sane mind, and entitled to be restored to her liberty.

Lastly. The said S. Gaitskell, though confined against her will as above represented, has at all times declared herself to be perfectly satisfied with the treatment she receives from Doctor Perfect, as to her diet, attendance, etc.

Unfortunately, the records are silent on the outcome of this case.

There were certainly some patients who lived for years in the madhouse — the larger it became, the more rooms were available for long-term use, and Perfect's establishment was used for the confinement of at least one lunatic criminal. Macalpine and Hunter, in their book *George III and the Mad Business*, comment that 'Strange to say, the treatment of the lunatic by the courts of Georgian England was often more merciful than that meted out by doctors and keepers'. Insane offenders were sometimes confined in madhouses without being brought to trial: in 1796, for example, a coroner's court sent Charles Lamb's sister, Mary, to the madhouse at Hoxton for murdering her mother while suffering from temporary insanity. Hunter and Macalpine note that in 1777 William Perfect's madhouse received a lunatic who was sent there for life for matricide. Others, too, a few of them perhaps no more than simple, were destined to spend their lives there. The parish register of West Malling records the burial in 1839, from what was by then known as the Lunatic Asylum, of Henry Mountfort, with the brief remark added by the vicar that 'He was an inoffensive, amiable man, much respected in the neighbourhood, and was an inmate of the asylum 32 years'.

Other burials of inmates of Perfect's establishment, noted as such in the parish register, are as follows:

1781 Mrs Mary Butcher
1782 Edward Nightingale
1783 Mrs Elizabeth Wait
     Alice Jaynes
1793 Hugh Norris, esq.
1795 Sarah Graham
1798 Mr Thomas Pilcher
1800 Anne Histead
1801 Mr Archibald Duff
1807 Mrs Anne East

In 1783, from being simply a surgeon, William Perfect had become an MD. An announcement in the *Kentish Gazette* informed the world that he had passed an examination to practise as a physician. Perfect's degree, however, was obtained from St Andrews, where it is known that such degrees could be bought. But it is possible that certain questions were put to those who applied for them, which might be construed as an examination; and certainly there can be little doubt that by then Perfect's skill, knowledge and experience entitled him to the honour.

He appears to have trained two of his sons to follow in his footsteps as surgeons, although they were never formally apprenticed, either to him or to any other doctor. Both were sons of his first marriage. William, the eldest son, born in 1758, practised as a surgeon at Wandsworth, where he is found taking an apprentice (for a premium of £100) in 1787, and another (for a premium of double that figure) in 1801. George, the third son, who was four years William's junior, was to stay in West Malling, where he became his father's assistant and close colleague. He, too, joined the freemasons, and both father and son appear to have been founder members of the Benevolent Society for the Relief of Widows and Orphans of Medical Men in the County of Kent, instituted in 1787: both were certainly members by 1790, and in 1809, the year of his father's death, George was acting as one of the Society's eight stewards for the western division of the county.

William Perfect's circumstances seem to have improved considerably in the eighties, as his reputation grew. In 1790 he was able to buy another house, a much larger one, with a yearly rental of £14 or £15, which would seem to have been fitted up additionally for his patients. Five years later he was paying rates on yet another property, of a similar size. All his properties were in Town Malling itself, however, and it was not until after the death of George Perfect, in 1821, that the asylum, now run by Robert Rix, moved into the larger premises of Malling Place.

During his lifetime William Perfect was successful in keeping competition at bay, no doubt due to the reputation which he had built up. In October 1784 a Mr Brigden ventured into the columns of the *Kentish Gazette* to advertise his lunatic asylum at Bethnal Green, where ladies and gentlemen could be

> Accommodated with board, washing and lodging etc., under the inspection of Mr Brigden, apothecary and man-midwife, whose approved medicine needs no other comment than the reputation it has gained in insanity, hysterical, hypochondriacal and epileptic complaints.

Mr Brigden emphasised his tender regard for his patients' different dispositions, and the need for a well-regulated diet in restoring respectable characters 'from wild fixed madness to cool sense and rational judgment' — words which are an almost direct quotation from Charles Seymour's 1776 eulogy of William Perfect! Brigden also offered to take into his house 'ladies subject to insanity during the latter period of pregnancy'.

Such an atttempt to lure the insane of Kent away from its own well established institution could not be overlooked by its founder, and an answering advertisement was placed in the *Kentish Gazette* by Perfect the following month. One is happy to see that he coolly dismisses Brigden's attempt to equate insanity and the discomforts of pregnancy!

> Lunatic Asylum. — Ladies and gentlemen continue to be accommo-
> dated with board, lodging, washing, etc. under the immediate
> inspection of Doctor Perfect, the sole proprietor and medical
> professor (an advantage of the utmost consequence, and which too
> seldom occurs!) whose approved medicines need no other comment
> than the reputation they have for many years gained in insanity, the
> epilepsy, hysteric passion, hypochondriac affection, and nervous
> complaints. His patients are treated with tenderness, delicacy,
> sympathising humanity, and a well-regulated diet.
>
> ... A generous attention to the situation of the fair sex in every
> stage of pregnancy, and particularly the last, if accompanied with
> symptoms of insanity (happily however a very rare instance) induces
> Doctor Perfect to recommend their own houses, at that critical
> period, as their safest and most proper residence.

It may have been the appearance of this competition which moved Perfect to renew his *Address to the Public* on the subject of insanity, which is here mentioned as 'this day published'. The same advertisement announces that the second edition of his book on insanity, here called *Cases of Insanity*, is now available, and that the second edition of *Cases in Midwifery* is to be published on 10 November of that year.

Real competition in the neighbourhood did not appear until 1792, when a Sussex doctor, Samuel Newington, opened a large and prestigious establishment just outside Ticehurst. In terms of size, Perfect's much more modest house (or rather, houses) had nothing to set against Ticehurst, with its pleasure grounds, aviary, moss-house and vineyard, but his established reputation clearly carried the day, and it was not until some years after his death that it was found necessary, if the Malling asylum was to continue, to transfer it to bigger premises.

London, in the meantime, offered an enlarged sphere of activity. William Perfect had become a member of the prestigious London Medical Society by 1795, and he seems to have set up a consultancy in London around the same time. A notice in the *Kentish Gazette* for 30 September 1796 states that he can be contacted at No.91 in the Strand, although without giving any days or hours. A Perfect presence seems to have been maintained there, because after his father's death, in 1809, George announced in the county papers (and presumably also in the London ones) that he himself was to be consulted 'at the Angel inn, behind St Clement's church, in the Strand, where he attends the first Monday and Tuesday in every month, from the hour of 10 o'clock in the morning till three in the afternoon'. It is probable that George, by then, had already been acting in place of his father for some time.

The Strand consultancy was probably a logical step for someone who had retained links with the capital since his apprenticeship days, visiting friends and using publishers there, and eventually seeing several of his children settled in and around London. A visit to town could be a mixed experience, however: in the winter of 1798 Mrs Perfect, who must sometimes have accompanied her husband, had the misfortune to lose a trunk, which was cut from the back of a postchaise as it stood outside her lodgings.

It is impossible to know the extent to which the ever-present atmosphere of madness may have thrown a shadow over the lives of William Perfect's children. In the later years, it is true, the insane were housed separately: an advertisement inserted in the *Maidstone Journal* by George Perfect a few weeks after his father's death mentions that epileptic and hypochondriac patients are accommodated in the family, separately from the licensed house, the plan probably established by his father. During the time his children were growing up, however, all the patients appear to have been accommodated in the Perfect house, alongside the doctor's family. Only Almeria, Perfect's youngest child, is known to have registered a protest, deliberately cutting her name on the window of her room one cold wintry afternoon, 15 January 1796, dangerously chipping out tiny splinters of glass. But her action may simply have been inspired by boredom, by pique at having been sent up to her room, or by a child's curiosity, wanting to see whether one of her father's medical instruments was sharp enough to cut glass.

Father and daughter:

William Perfect's signature to a 1780 vestry meeting in connection with the rebuilding of West Malling church, when he served as a member of the supervisory committee.

Almeria's name scratched on the window of her room.

Chapter 6

Finale

The short-lived *Freemasons' Magazine* of the 1790s offered another outlet for the verse which William Perfect continued to enjoy writing. It also, in October 1796, reviewed a new collection which he had brought out, the title of which, *Poetic Effusions*, was a mild pun on the medical and literary background of the author. *Poetic Effusions, Pastoral, Moral, Amatory and Descriptive* probably made few claims to originality, although its editor, in his Preface, found in it a 'constancy to nature' which had, indeed, always been one of Perfect's hallmarks as a writer. The proceeds of a second edition, brought out by Perfect in 1799, and advertised in the *Maidstone Journal* in September of that year, were intended for the relief of 'a worthy but indigent character'.

It is the *Freemasons' Magazine* which, as well as a portrait of William Perfect as a young man, gives us the fullest contemporary description of him. The 'Memoirs of William Perfect MD, Member of the London Medical Society, and Provincial Grand Master of the Masons for the County of Kent' opened the issue for September 1795, and were obviously written shortly after he had been elevated to the highest post in Kentish freemasonry. They are useful in extending our knowledge of Perfect's output. In particular, they refer to a 1791 publication, *A Remarkable Case of Madness*, which apparently dealt with the insanity of an eleven-year-old, and to some 'moral, religious and instructive letters which he has written and published with considerable success'.

Perfect's achievements in the medical, literary and masonic fields are outlined, reference is made to his ready charity towards the needy, and the writer hopes that he 'who never suffers the whispers of vanity to approach his ear' will not be offended by what has been said. Nevertheless, a certain tenderness towards his professional reputation is apparent in the date assigned here to his book on insanity: the revised edition of 1787, dedicated to the founder of the London Medical Society, John Coakley Lettsom, (although here dated even later, to 1790) is said to be the book's first appearance, thus suppressing all mention of the first two unrevised editions of *Methods of Cure* — and, it has to be said, adding fuel to the theory that this was first intended purely as a publicity brochure. *Cases in Midwifery*, of 1781-3, which remained unchanged throughout its three editions, is here, somewhat curiously, dated to 1787, the year after the third edition had appeared.

Was this vanity? Maybe it is unfair to pursue an advertising puff with a bibliographer's zeal: *Methods of Cure* turned out to be a template; it could just as easily have disappeared as an ephemera, and it is perhaps doing William Perfect an injustice to insist on 'first edition' status for something which was intended as no such thing.

Overall, the writer gives a candid picture of his subject, hinting at criticism and even – dare one say it – ridicule: 'Dr Perfect, in the cultivation of his genius, has not escaped the shafts of criticism', and 'Dr Perfect ... lives as much beloved by his acquaintance as perhaps any gentleman in the kingdom, and as much respected by *all those who know him best*' (sic). Did he sometimes appear too rigidly upright, with an almost naive belief in the possibility of one man embodying all the virtues? From such a belief in his father, as epitomised in several of his poems and given more lengthy substance in the opening lines of the 'Memoirs', he seems to have gone on to hope that he, too, might be such a man. Certainly he was someone who believed in himself. This is apparent, for example, in the diction of some of his poems, and the ease with which he mints new words when he needs them. It was an innocent stance, yet it may on occasion have proved difficult to live with for those nearest to him.

The 'Memoirs' were clearly written in consultation with William Perfect, otherwise it seems unlikely that the writer would have known of works on which Perfect was engaged but which were not, in the event, ever to appear: a 'Symptomatology' – intended, perhaps, to be his magnum opus – and an 'Essay on the Epilepsy'. Nevertheless, the writer makes an independent judgment of his subject, concluding finally that he has 'abilities that should command general respect, and virtues that are entitled to universal esteem'. It seems a measured judgment, and well earnt by someone whose ideals were set even higher: William Perfect bore a difficult name.

It is probably a tribute to Perfect's care and attention as a father that his nine surviving children would seem to have grown up quite normally. At the time of their father's death, in 1809, all were married, or had been married, with the exception of Lucy, and most of them had children. William and Thomas had lost their first wives – and William his second also. Elizabeth, the eldest daughter, had married Henry Stratford, and by 1809 was already a grandmother. Sarah had married the painter, engraver and publisher, Sylvester Harding, and in 1809 they were living in Pall Mall, although Sylvester was to outlive his father-in-law by only a few months. Folliott, in 1791, had married the fourth son of a former governor of Madras, Charles Wynch, of Henley Castle in Worcestershire, but by 1805 she had been widowed and in January of that year, in what appears to have been a joint wedding ceremony, had married Captain Thomas Young of the Royal Marine Corps at the same time that her youngest sister, Almeria, was married to his brother, Lieutenant E. S. Young, of the Chatham Division of Royal Marines.

Of Henrietta, William Perfect's rattle-tongued second wife, we know little. She died early in 1804, after a long illness, at the age of 58, and Perfect was to marry for a third time in or around 1805, taking for his bride a second Elizabeth, some thirty years his junior, who was almost certainly Elizabeth Selby, and a member of a prominent West Malling family. But their time together was to be very short. Although ill in the summer of 1805, Perfect seems to have recovered sufficiently to carry out some of his duties as Provincial Grand Master of the Kent masons the following year, but by February 1808, when he made his will, although able to describe himself as 'being in a tolerable good state of health and of sound and disposing mind, memory and understanding', he was perhaps already aware, as a doctor, that he had not long to live. Two codicils, added in April and May 1809, were signed by him with a mark only, and he was to breathe his last at the beginning of the following month.

As he had requested in his will, his body was interred, in a triple coffin of oak, lead and oak respectively, in the vault at East Malling which he had himself had made some years earlier to receive the remains of his father and grandfather. The funeral, as he had wished it, was held at night, the cortege, of hearse, three coaches and one private carriage, setting out from West Malling by torchlight. After the service an address was given to those assembled by Dr Thompson of Rochester, Deputy Provincial Grand Master. The inscription on the chest tomb over the vault, 'To the beloved memory of William Perfect', now virtually illegible, was to record that he,

> after a life spent in the arduous duties of his profession, adorned with literary taste, and softened by the emotions of a heart which glowed for others' good, exchanged it for immortality June 5th 1809.

By then George had probably been running the 'mad business' for several years, although it was only legally made over to him on William Perfect's death. Under the terms of the will, George was left the building 'situate near the High Street in West Malling', with all its fixtures and fittings, together with all Perfect's 'business and profession of insanity'.

To him, too, went all William Perfect's books on medical, surgical and obstetric subjects, his electrical machine and surgical instruments, as well as £100 sterling and a few smaller items, including the doctor's masonic seal and his large pair of Spanish pistols. Nevertheless, George did not become a second William Perfect, and it was due to his insolvency in 1815 that the asylum passed into other hands.

Bequests to the other children followed, largely in the form of money or of interest from stocks in the East India Company. Lucy, as well as a bequest of this kind, was left the bed, with its furnishings and hangings, and all the furniture, in the best bedroom in the house her father had been renting from William Scatton in West Malling. Almeria, whose bequest of interest from East India stock was similar to that of Lucy's, also received £150 and her father's part in a tontine, described as 'the tontine of Mr O'Hara', as well as 'my pianoforte, my large silver teapot, silver fish slice, silver gravy spoon and silver salad spoon, and my portrait by Sylvester Harding'. William Perfect's many books were distributed between several members of the family, including his wife Elizabeth, who was left 'one hundred and fifty books of her own selection', and a book-case in which to put them. Elizabeth and Sarah, the two daughters of Perfect's first wife, both received monetary bequests, and, touchingly, china bowls and mugs which had belonged to their mother. To Elizabeth, too, went 'my large silver tankard'. It had become a very large family, with over thirty grandchildren, but William Perfect seems to have tried to remember everyone. Nephews Thomas and John Skerrett each received twenty pounds, and the will reveals other relatives, a Mrs Eleanor Rathwell of Bath, widow, and a widowed niece, Mrs Frances Frisby of Sandwich. William Perfect's servants, Samuel and Jane Kidwell, were to receive a year's wages, over and above what was due to them at the time of his death, and they, and all his other servants, who had been in his employ for at least a year prior to his death, were to be provided with a good suit of mourning. A masonic charitable institution, the Royal Cumberland School, was left £50. The executors were named as his two sons George and Thomas, and William Moore, druggist, of Fleet Street, who must have been a friend of his later years.

The two codicils made only a few minor adjustments to his will, providing for the altered state of some property, which Perfect had originally left in trust to be sold by his executors, but which by the time of his death he had himself already sold, and adding a few small bequests for friends. James Selby of West Malling was left ten guineas for mourning and two guineas for a ring, and the same sum for a mourning ring was also left to Richard Thompson esq., of Rochester, Thomas Killick of Gravesend, Samuel Clanfield, a broker on the stock exchange, Thomas Assiter, a stone mason of Maidstone, Robert Richard, an organist, also of Maidstone, Dr Robert Caton, who was perhaps the doctor who had charge of him during his final months, and Matthew Garland, senior, of Deptford.

Garland, the Deptford shipwright, who had risen in freemasonry to hold the office formerly filled by Perfect himself, that of Provincial Grand Orator, was perhaps gifted in a similar way to William Perfect, a man of arts as well as of science; and the rather fine 'Elegy on the death of W. Perfect MD, late Right Worshipful Provincial Grand Master', quoted by Sydney Pope, although unattributed, seems likely to have come from the pen of Matthew Garland, who had been a very close friend. It describes the doctor as well as the freemason, the man of science and the Enlightenment as well as the man of feeling, and a few lines from it seem to offer a fitting conclusion to this life of William Perfect of West Malling.

'Twas thine with eloquence and mental powers
To give delight through captivating hours;
Or when the Muse with radiant beauty glowed,
Witness 'The Months', how sweet thy numbers flowed!
If on hilarity thy mind was bent
What could excel 'The Lodge within the Tent'?
Or, did thine all-creating fancy stray
To Preston Court, the Park, or Beltenge Bay,
Nature and Genius took thee by each hand —
Climate and seasons were at thy command.

When festive customs called thee to appear,
The Sons of Science hailed the rising year.
Order and Moral Conduct led the way,
And thy superior talent crowned the day.
No austere rules were thine, no distant pride,
At once politely free and dignified,
The annual fete was, under thy control,
'The feast of reason and the flow of soul';
Where kind benevolence, with fostering hand
And sentimental honours took their stand.

To these bright parts, instructively were joined
A hand and heart beneficent and kind.
Humanity through all thy actions shone,
And in thy breast compassion held her throne.

Professional repute, so justly due,
With marked distinction was conferred on you.
Debilitated reason felt thy power;
Great was thy skill in nature's trying hour:
Gentle (not timorous) when danger called,
Howe'er the human frame might be enthralled.

May honest fervour compensation make
For want of genius, and for friendship's sake,
Yes, generous friendship, disinterested, free,
Bestowed by Kent's masonic chief on me;
For this concession let me in return
Strew grateful incense o'er the donor's urn.

Sources and Bibliography

Works by William Perfect

A Bavin of Bays (London, 1763)

An Elegy on a Storm which happened in West Kent on the 13th of August 1763 (London, 1764)

Calumny Dissected (advertised, price 2s., 1764; not traced)

The Laurel Wreath (2 vols., London, 1766)

An Address to the Public, on the Subject of Insanity (?1778; reprinted 1784)

Methods of Cure, in Some Particular Cases of Insanity: the Epilepsy, Hypochondriacal Affection, Hysteric Passion, and Nervous Disorders (Rochester, ?1778)

— 2nd edition, enlarged, and entitled *Cases of Insanity, the Epilepsy, Hypochondriacal Affection, Hysteric Passion, and Nervous Disorders, Successfully Treated* (Rochester, n.d., but advertised June 1783)

— 3rd edition, revised, and entitled *Select Cases in the Different Species of Insanity, Lunacy or Madness* (Rochester, 1787)

— 4th edition, entitled *Annals of Insanity* (London, 1801)

— ?7th edition, (1809)

Cases in Midwifery (2 vols., Rochester, ?1781-1783)

— 2nd edition (Rochester, 1784)

— 3rd edition (Rochester, 1787)

A Remarkable Case of Madness (1791; not traced)

Poetic Effusions (reviewed, price 2s.6d., 1796; not traced)

— 2nd edition (advertised, price 3s.6d., 1799; not traced)

'Appearances upon opening the body of a woman, who died the beginning of August 1762, after eating a large quantity of cucumbers', in *The Medical Museum*, Vol.1, 1763, 212-3

'An attempt to improve medical prognostication', in *The Medical Museum*, Vol.3, 1764, 287-312

Poems in *The Weeds of Parnassus* (ed. Folly Streeter; not traced)

Journalism (poetry and prose) in the following:

Freemasons' Magazine

General Magazine of Arts and Sciences

Gentleman's Magazine

Kentish Gazette

Martin's Magazine

Mechell's Political Chronicle

St James' Evening Post

St James' Chronicle

Sentimental Magazine

Universal Magazine

Westminster Journal

Record and Manuscript Sources

Bromley Local Studies Library
P47/1/29 SS Peter and Paul, Bromley: Burial Register 1678-1778

British Library Newspaper Library, Colindale
Kentish Gazette, 1768-1809
Kentish Post, 1757-1768
Maidstone Journal, 1786-1809

Centre for Kentish Studies, Maidstone
P243/1/1 St Mary, West Malling: Burial Register 1690-1817
P243/4/1 West Malling church rates 1700-1787
Q/SB/1770 Apprenticeship of Pury Samuel Caister to William Perfect

Q/SMaW9,10,11,12   William Perfect's madhouse licences
TR2270/1   Photograph of Almeria's name scratched on glass
at 104 High Street, West Malling

Masonic Museum and Library, Canterbury
  William Perfect MSS
  Spiller, R.A., 'William Perfect MD of West Malling, Kent,
  1737-1809: Provincial Grand Master of Kent 1795-1809'

Public Record Office, Kew
  IR/1/18   Duty paid on apprentices

Bibliography

Copywell, J. *The Shrubs of Parnassus* (1760)

French, C.N. *The Story of St Luke's Hospital* (1951)

Gaudron, A.W. *Concision and Precision: Poems for Fred* (Australia, 1993)

The Gentleman's Magazine, 1745-1809

Holworthy, F.M.R. 'Bromley College Register, 1679-1800', *The Pedigree Register*, Vol.2, Nos.21-23 (1912)

Hunter, R. and MacAlpine, I. *Three Hundred Years of Psychiatry*, 1535-1860 (1963)

Lane, J. 'The Medical Practitioners of Provincial England in 1783', *Medical History*, 28 (1984), 353-371

Loudon, I. *Medical Care and the General Practitioner 1750-1850* (Oxford, 1986)

MacAlpine, I. and Hunter, R. *George III and the Mad-Business* (1969)

Mackenzie, C., *Psychiatry for the Rich. A History of Ticehurst Private Asylum, 1792-1917* (1992)

The Medical Museum, Vols.1-4 (1763-176?7; reprinted 1781)

The Medical Register (1779; 1780; 1783)

'Memoirs of William Perfect M.D., Member of the London Medical Society, and Provincial Grand Master of the Masons for the County of Kent', *Freemasons' Magazine*, Vol.5 (July-Dec, 1795), 147-151

Pope, Sydney 'Freemasonry in Canterbury and Provincial Grand Lodge, 1785-1809, and Dr Perfect, Provincial Grand Master of Kent, 1795-1809', *Ars Quatuor Coronatorum*, Vol.52 (1939), 6-58

Razzell, P. *The Conquest of Smallpox: The Impact of Inoculation on Smallpox Mortality in Eighteenth Century Britain* (Firle, 1977)

Seymour, C. *A New Topographical, Historical and Commercial Survey of the Cities, Towns and Villages of the County of Kent* (Canterbury, 1776)

Spencer, H.R. *History of British Midwifery from 1650 to 1800* (1927)

Streeter, F. *Hampton Court* (Rochester, 1778)

Wallis, P.J. and Wallis, R.V. *Eighteenth Century Medics* (2nd edition, Newcastle upon Tyne, 1988)

Index

C

D

E